The Nutrient Bible

EIGHTH EDITION

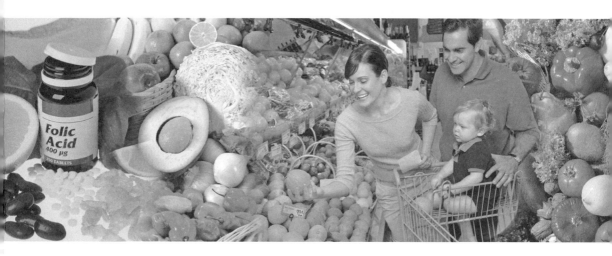

Henry Osiecki

The Nutrient Bible © Henry Osiecki.

All rights reserved. Used by Permission.

8th Edition

The Moral right of the author has been asserted.

For more Information, please contact:

BIO CONCEPTS PUBLISHING

Unit 9, 783 Kingsford Smith Drive
EAGLE FARM QLD 4009 AUSTRALIA
info@bioconcepts.com.au

National Library of Australia
Cataloguing-in-Publication data:

Osiecki, Henry.
The Nutrient Bible

8th edition
ISBN 978-1-875239-53-5

Book Publishing Services Provided by:
AG Publishing
Email: info@agpublishing.com
Website: www.agpublishing.com

Design: Debbie Elliott

Presentation of data

The vitamins, amino acids, minerals, contingent nutrients and accessory food extracts chosen for coverage in this book are those that have the widest acceptance by the various researchers in these fields. I have used the vitamin definition as formulated by R.J. Klutsky as my guide -

"A vitamin is defined as a biologically active organic compound, a controlling agent essential for normal health and growth (its absence causing a deficiency disease or disorder) **not synthesized** within the body, available in the diet in small amounts, and carried in the circulatory system in small concentrations to act on target organs or tissue".

I have added a new category called contingent nutrient that are normally not considered in nutritional texts.

The definition of a contingent nutrient is -

"A biologically active, organic compound, a controlling agent essential for normal homeostasis, health and growth (its absence causing deficiency, disease or disorder) **synthesized within the body** but not in sufficient quantity to meet the demands of the body due to heredity, aging, stress, or disease."

Examples of this are: carnitine and other non-essential amino acids, glucosamine, carnosine, r-lipoic acid, nicotinamide adenine dinucleotide (NAD), phosphatidyl serine, glutathione and many others.

Accessory food extracts or bio-factors also play a considerable role in maintaining optimum health and have been included. Nutrient factors such as: isoflavones, fibre, mucopolysaccharides, digestive enzymes and probiotics, are some of the accessory biofactors described.

Metabolic Individuality and RDA

The subject of nutrient requirements needs comment. There is now sufficient evidence to indicate that the concept of biological individuality has much merit. This genetic diversity within the human population is expressed nutritionally by variations in absorption, excretion and metabolism of nutrients, resulting in significant differences in nutritional requirements. Thus, the recommended daily allowance (RDA) as stated in this book, should be considered only as an average figure, and variations (increase or decrease) of twenty fold or more in individual human requirements may be found, depending on the genetic and physiological state of the individual. The supplementary range (SR) given is the safe therapeutic dose for a range of disease states mentioned.

Factors increasing demand:

This section lists drugs, chemicals, disease states or conditions that are likely to increase the need for the nutrient.

Function facilitated:

This section lists the physiological function that the nutrient may play a role in.

Deficiency may cause or be associated with:

Deficiency symptoms are listed, as well as conditions that are associated with deficiency. The symptoms listed are not only of deficiency states but also include physiological states that contribute to the deficiency state.

A deficiency of a nutrient can occur if the body excretes more of a particular nutrient than normal, or if it cannot absorb the nutrient properly or if it is not provided in the diet. This is called an absolute deficiency.

A relative deficiency can occur when cells metabolise or excrete a particular nutrient faster than other nutrients associated in a particular biochemical pathway, resulting in alteration in the ratio between these nutrients. This causes the altering of their delicate balance or activity.

Therapeutic Uses:

Lists the conditions that are responsive to, as well as those that have an increased need for, the nutrient. These will include the classical deficiency diseases, but also health conditions that may respond to the nutrient.

Synergistic Nutrients

Lists nutrients that work together in particular metabolic pathways as well as cofactors that activate the nutrient in question. Supplementing with synergistic combination of nutrients with the nutrient in question will result in better health outcomes at lower dose of the star nutrient for a condition.

Vitamins are closely associated with the metabolic function of minerals. For instance, zinc is required to mobilise vitamin A from body stores. If zinc is deficient, a person may have sufficient stores of vitamin A in the liver and still have signs of vitamin A deficiency e.g. night blindness. Vitamin A supplementation will not have any effect on this condition unless zinc status is restored.

It must be noted that synergistic nutrients at high doses can be antagonistic to the particular nutrient that is being supported. If this occurs, a relative deficiency of that particular nutrient may occur. Eg excess calcium can reduce the activity of magnesium or excess zinc intake can increase the secretion of copper.

Drug/Nutrient Interactions

A drug/nutrient interaction is viewed a as physical, physiologic or pathological relationship between a drug and nutrient and the nutritional status of the individual. An interaction is considered significant from a clinical perspective if it alters a therapeutic response or compromises the nutritional status. The risk of experiencing a significant interaction is determined by a number of factors:

- The nutritional status of the individual
- The presence of chronic disease associated with multi drug- use
- The age of the person, particularly at each end of the spectrum
- Genetic influences associated with variant drug metabolism
- Impaired organ function
- Imbalances in the nutrient requirement and intake

I have tried to be inclusive of these factors when considering which nutrient interacts with a particular drug.

References have not been included to save space and make the book easier to use. However, for those who require reference material, I suggest going on pub med and do a search on a particular nutrient. Eg nutrient (in question) + function or nutrient + deficiency state or disease or drug, nutrient + metabolism or toxicity etc.

Or

Werbach MR, MD. *Nutritional Influences on Illness. 2nd edition.* 1996; Third Line Press: California.

Osiecki H. *The Physician's Handbook of Clinical Nutrition. 7th edition.* 2006; Bio concepts Publishing: Australia.

I would recommend the following journals, which have significant information on nutrients:

Medical Hypothesis
Lancet
International Clinical Nutritional Reviews
Annual Review of Nutrition
Annual Review of Biochemistry
International Journal for Vitamin and Nutrition Research.

Henry Osiecki

BSc.(Hons), Post Graduate Dip.Nutrition & Dietetics

Author's Note – Diagrams

All diagrams included in this book have been drawn in Adobe Illustrator CS2.

DISCLAIMER

Legal & Medical Disclaimer

Patients with particular medical conditions should consult their physicians before beginning any nutritional program. **This book is not intended to be a substitute for medical care or advice.** Any of the recommendations made in this book must be used under the guidance of a qualified health practitioner. Dosages are meant to be used as guidelines only and may vary according to the specific needs of each individual.

Contents

CHAPTER 3   MINERALS

CHAPTER 4   CONTINGENT NUTRIENT FACTORS
Enzymes and Miscellaneous Factors

CHAPTER 5   TOXIC METALS

CHAPTER 6   DISEASE & NUTRIENT REQUIREMENTS

CHAPTER 1

Vitamins

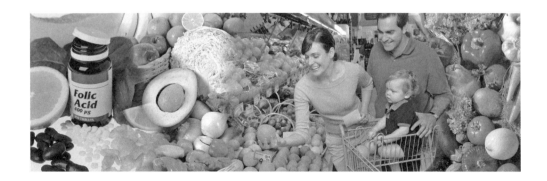

Vitamin A

Retinol, retinal, retinoic acid, precursor – beta-carotene

SOURCE

Apricots, barley grass, butter, carrots, egg yolk, fish liver oils (cod, salmon, and halibut), green leafy vegetables, hard & cream cheese, kohlrabi, liver, mint, spinach, sweet potatoes.

PROCESSING LOSSES

Heating vegetables (green, yellow) 15-35%

FACTORS INCREASING DEMAND

Air pollution, alcohol, athletes, autism, cancer, chlordane exposure, copper and cadmium toxicity, cystic fibrosis, DDT, diabetics, diarrhoea, dieldrin, fat intolerance, gall and pancreatic disease, giardiasis, infection, protein-energy malnutrition, smoking, stress.

FUNCTIONS FACILITATED

Activates T and B lymphocytes, lipid antioxidant, adrenocorticoid and steroid hormone synthesis, bone growth, controls gene expression, differentiates leukemic cells and possibly induces apoptosis, enhances adhesion between cells and restores contact inhibition of growth, increases resistance to infection – enhances phagocytes and antibody production, increases iron utilization for haemoglobin formation, maintains gap function between cells, maintains lysosome stability and mucosal barrier to infection, maintenance of the myelin sheath, membrane integrity, mucopolysaccharide synthesis, vision, visual purple synthesis, protects against epithelial carcinogenesis, reduces buccal cancer in betel nut and tobacco chewers, stimulates neurotrophic factor synthesis (GDNF).

Supports hippocampal retinoid receptor pathways that are critically involved in: vision, sensory perception, language processing and attention.

DEFICIENCY MAY CAUSE OR BE ASSOCIATED WITH:

Acne, allergies, bone loss, Bitot's spots, corneal ulceration, cysts on endocrine and other glands, decrease in function of neutrophils and natural killer cells, decrease in corticosteroid production, decreased tearing, diabetes type I, diminishes antibody response of TH2 cells, dry hair, easily breaking finger nails, epithelial cancers (lung, colon, breast, prostate), hyperkeratosis, increased morbidity and mortality in young children, inflammation of the eye, involution of the thymus gland, keratomalacia, nephritis, night blindness, perifollicular hyperkeratosis, poor bone growth, poor immunity, poor sense of taste and smell, retardation of growth, rigid finger nails, rough dry skin, skin cancer, sinus problems, tinnitus, weight loss, xerophthalmia, xerosis.

THERAPEUTIC USES

Acne (rosacea and vulgaris), acute leukemia, AIDS, arthritis, asthma, autism, benzo-alpha pyrene exposure, bronchitis, cancer, cataract prevention, cervical dysplasia, coeliac disease, colds, conjunctivitis, Crohn's disease, cystitis, diabetes, diarrhoea, diseases of connective tissues, dry skin, dyslexia, eczema, eye irritation, fibro cystic breast disease, gut trauma, heavy menstrual bleeding, Hodgkin's disease, inflammatory bowel disorder, kerotomalacia, liver detoxification, measles, multiple sclerosis, night blindness, optic neuritis, pancreatic and gall bladder disease, pollution exposure, poor immunity, psoriasis, pulmonary emphysema, pruitis, retinitis pigmentosa, tinnitus, tooth and gum disorders, tumours, ulcers (duodenal and gastric), ulcerative colitis, viral infections, viral meningitis, wound healing, xerophthalmia (dry eyes).

DAILY DOSAGE

Adults RDA	5,000-9,000 IU
SR	10,000-50,000 IU (as retinol palmitate for a few days)
Infants	<1,500 IU
Children	<2,500 IU
Pregnancy	<5,000 IU/day – as it is associated with birth defects

RDA by age in Retinol Equivalents

(Note: 1 IU = 0.300 µg retinol):

Infant	375 µg
1 - 3 yrs	400 µg
4 - 6 yrs	500 µg
7 - 10 yrs	700 µg
Adult Male	1000 µg
Adult Female	800 µg
Lactation	1200-1300 µg
Plasma deficiency levels	<10µg/l or 0.35 mmol/l

High doses should not be taken for prolonged periods of time.

Dosage required to produce toxicity is highly variable. Chronic toxicity can occur from dosages of 26,000 IU to 1,000,000 IU/day for 2 years. As it is a fat-soluble vitamin, it can accumulate in the body over time. It is imperative that high doses should not be taken over a prolonged period of time.

EFFECTS OF OVERDOSAGE AND TOXICITY

> 75,000 IU/day
Exophthalmia, fatigue, headache, hypercalcaemia, hypercalcuria, increased cerebrospinal pressure, insomnia, irritability, nausea, nerve lesions, painful bones and joints, peeling skin. High intake of Vitamin A during pregnancy may cause birth defects.

Chronic effects
Abnormal bone growth, amenorrhoea, anorexia, birth defects, bone (at doses 10 times RDA) and muscle pain, headache, increased blood lipids, irritability, itching, jaundice, loss of hair. Vitamin D and glucaric acid reduce retinoid toxicity.

Vitamin D may mitigate some of the toxic effects of Vitamin A.

TECHNICAL NOTES

SYNERGISTIC NUTRIENTS
Vitamin B_2, B_3, B_{12}, C, D, E, magnesium, selenium, manganese, potassium, phosphorus, carotenoids, iodine, tyrosine, zinc.

DRUG/NUTRIENT INTERACTIONS

Decrease vitamin A absorption:
  Bile acid sequestrants – cholestyramine, colestipol, colesevelam
  Neomycin

Decrease body or tissue levels of vitamin A:
  Orlistat, Corticosteroid medications – prednisone, hydrocortisone, methylprednisolone, prednisolone, betamethasone, budesonide, triamcinolone, dexamethasone, cortisone, beclomethasone, flunisolide, fluticasone, fludrocortisone, mometasone

Increase toxicity of vitamin A:

Vitamin A derivatives – isotretinoin, tretinoin, acitretin, alitretinoin

Reduce vitamin A status:

Oral contraceptives – norethindrone, ethynodiol diacetate, norgestrel, norgestimate, ethinyl estradiol, drospirenone, desogestrel, levonorgestrel

Bromobenzene, phenobarbital, sodium benzoate.

NUTRIENT/NUTRIENT INTERACTIONS

Large oral doses of **vitamin A** decrease the absorption of **vitamin E** into the body.

TARGET TISSUES

Adrenals, bone, germinal epithelium, intestines, liver, retina, salivary glands, skin.

ENZYME SYSTEMS INVOLVED

- Hydroxylating deoxycorticosterone to corticosterone.
- Maintains stability of lysosomes & cell membranes.

Sulfurylases – (ATP + Sulphate → Phosphoadenosine phosphosulfate) required for mucopolysaccharide or glycoprotein synthesis.

DEFICIENCY SYMPTOMS AS RELATED TO METABOLIC ACTION

Bone development	Formation of chondroitin sulphate in cartilage.
Growth retardation	Effects on steroid synthesis, bone growth, and membrane structure.
Keratinisation	Effects on membranes and mucopolysaccharide biosynthesis.
Visual defects	Absence of retinene precursors.

Vitamin A deficiency may be viewed as a proliferative and immune disease. As it relates to all connective tissues, its effects extend via the basal membrane to all structures they coat – endothelia, mesothelia, and neuroglia.

Retinoic Acid and Vitamin D compete for the same nuclear receptor partners.

INTERNATIONAL UNITS CONVERSION

1 IU = 0.300 µg retinol
1 IU = 0.344 µg retinyl acetate
1 IU = 0.550 µg retinyl palmitate
1 IU = 0.359 µg retinyl propionate

STRUCTURE OF VITAMIN A

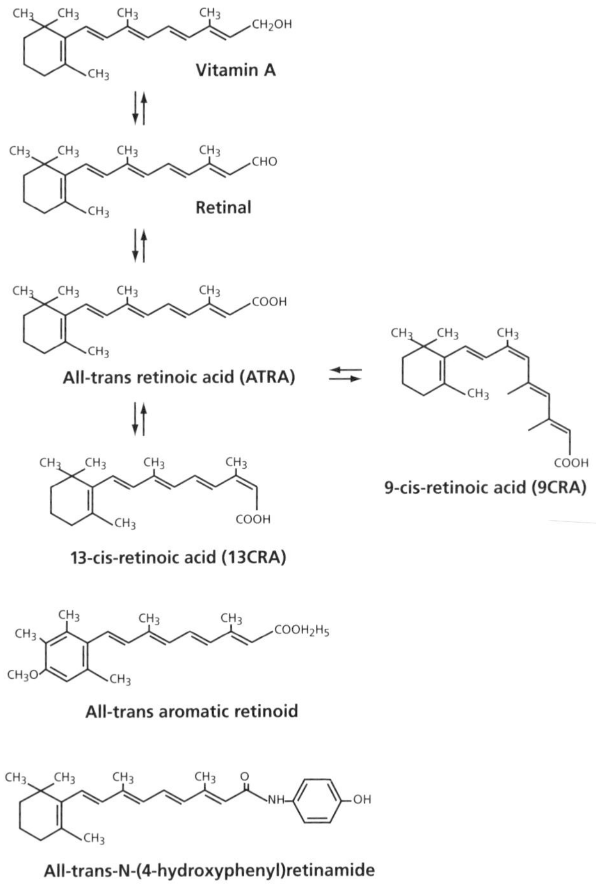

Vitamin A

Retinal

All-trans retinoic acid (ATRA)

9-cis-retinoic acid (9CRA)

13-cis-retinoic acid (13CRA)

All-trans aromatic retinoid

All-trans-N-(4-hydroxyphenyl)retinamide

Vitamin B1

Cocarboxylase; Active form – thiamine pyrophosphate (TPP)

SOURCE

Asparagus, beef, brewer's yeast, lamb, legumes, liver, nuts, pork, rye, spirulina, wheat germ, whole grains.

PROCESSING LOSSES

Unstable to heat and light

Meat roasting – 40-60%, milling of flour – 60-80%, baking bread – 5-15%, vegetable cooking – 60-80%

Sulphur dioxide and sulphite destroy vitamin B1, exposure of food to alkaline conditions (>pH 8)

FACTORS INCREASING DEMAND

Ageing, AIDS or HIV infection, athletes, autonomic dysfunction, Crohn's disease, diabetes, diarrhoea, eating disorders, excessive coffee, tea, alcohol, raw fish and sugar intake; alcohol withdrawal, excessive intake of blueberries and red cabbage, dialysis, fever, folate deficiency, formaldehyde exposure, gastrointestinal surgery, hyperactivity, hyperemesis gravidarum, hyperthyroidism, infection with *Bacillus thiaminolyticus*, lactation, lead poisoning, liver disease, malabsorption from pyloric stenosis, gastroenterostomy; metabolic disorders (subacute necrotizing encephalopathy, maple syrup urine disease, pyruvate carboxylase deficiency, hyperalaninemia); malaria, ulcerative colitis, dysentery, steatorrhoea, gastritis, pancreatitis or prolonged diarrhoea, parasitic infections, pregnancy, raw fish intake, excessive intake of refined food, smoking, stress, strenuous exercise, sulphite exposure, hyerthyroid disease.

FUNCTIONS FACILITATED

Acetyl-choline synthesis (Ach), appetite, cofactor in over 24 enzyme systems in the conversion of alpha keto acids to acyl ions, aldehydes and carboxylic acid i.e. decarboxylation of keto acids; cofactor of hexose mono-phosphate shunt – used by the adrenal cortex, leucocytes, red blood cells and breast tissue; central and peripheral nerve cell function, digestion, energy production, gastrointestinal tone, growth, mimics ACh in the brain, myocardial function, neuro-transmission, neutrophil motility, production of hydrochloric acid, converts pyruvate to acetyl CoA, regulates cell ion channels, sugar metabolism.

DEFICIENCY MAY CAUSE OR BE ASSOCIATED WITH:

Abdominal discomfort, absence of ankle jerk, anorexia, appetite loss, ataxia, autonomic dysfunction, backache, beriberi, burning feet, cardiac failure, cardiomeglia, calf muscle tenderness, chronic fatigue syndrome, congestive heart failure, constipation, decrease complement activity, decrease phagocytic activity of peripheral leucocytes, decrease antibody production, degeneration of axonal sheaths, difficulty rising from squatting position, difficulty in talking and swallowing, disruption of blood brain barrier, elevated blood pyruvate and lactate, fatigue, fluid retention, foot drop, glaucoma, gut disorders, hair loss, heart pain, hypotension, inability to concentrate, ion channel pathologies, insomnia, irritability, lactic acidosis, local cerebral hypoperfusion, loss of reflexes and vibratory sense, memory deficits, mental depression, moodiness, muscle weakness, nausea, nervous exhaustion, neuritis, neuromuscular disorders, numbness and tingling of hands and feet nystagmus, ophthalmoplegia, palpitations, paraesthesia, painful click of the knee, paralysis, peripheral neuropathy, poor muscular co-ordination, rapid pulse, retarded growth, shortness of breath, sleep disturbance, sore calf muscles, sweating, tachycardia, toe drop, toe and heal pain, unco-operativeness, weight loss, Wernicke's-Korsakoff Syndrome or psychosis, wide pulse pressure.

A deficiency of this vitamin causes the disease beriberi, in which the patient presents with muscle weakness, ataxia, footdrop, ophthalmoplegia, nystagmus, and neuropathy. Three forms of beriberi are: "wet" (edematous) or "dry" (nonedematous) and cerebral.

Dry beriberi refers to neuromuscular complications such as: peripheral neuropathy and weakness – burning feet, exaggerated reflexes, diminished sensation and weakness in the legs and arms, muscle pains, and ultimately seizures in severe cases.

Wet beriberi refers to cardiovascular complications such as: heart failure (Shoshin-type beriberi); cardiovascular complications such as: rapid heart rate, pulmonary edema (water in the lungs), and heart failure/cardiomyopathy (Shoshin-type beriberi).

Cerebral beriberi refers to central nervous system (brain) complications such as: Wernicke's encephalopathy (abnormal eye movements, stance/gait abnormalities, mental dysfunction) or Korsakoff's psychosis (apathy, confusion, severe memory deficits/amnesia, abnormal eye movements, stance/gait abnormalities, mental dysfunction), Korsakoff's psychosis (apathy, confusion, severe memory deficits/amnesia), or the combination of the two (Wernicke-Korsakoff syndrome).

Beriberi is regarded as a medical emergency because it can progress to cardiac failure.

THERAPEUTIC USES

AIDS, alcoholism, alcohol withdrawal, autonomic dysfunction, beriberi, burning feet, chronic fatigue syndrome, congestive heart failure, constipation, diabetes, diarrhoea, Down's Syndrome, the elderly, emotional instability, fearfulness with agitation, fevers, hyperactivity, hyperthyroidism, indigestion, irritability, lead poisoning, macrosomia (abnormal high body weight), memory deficits; metabolic genetic diseases – subacute necrotizing encephalopathy (SNE, Leigh's disease), maple syrup urine disease (branched-chain aminoacidopathy), and lactic acidosis associated with pyruvate carboxylase deficiency and hyperalaninemia; multiple sclerosis, neuritis, numbness in hands and feet, parasympathetic underactivity, peripheral neuropathy, poor appetite, poor immunity, pregnancy, poor appetite, sonophobia, toe and heal pain, Wernicke's encephalopathy, Korsakoff's psychosis, Wernicke-Korsakoff syndrome.

DAILY DOSAGE	
RDA	1-5 mg
SR	5-150 mg
Infant	0.5 mg
Children	0.7 mg

EFFECTS OF OVERDOSAGE AND TOXICITY
Dosages >125mg/kg
Nervousness, oedema, shortness of breath, sensation of heat, sweating, tachycardia, tremors.

TECHNICAL NOTES

SYNERGISTIC NUTRIENTS

Vitamin B_2, B_3, B_5, B_6, B_{12}, copper, choline, manganese magnesium, molybdenum, phosphate, zinc.

DRUG/NUTRIENT INTERACTIONS

Decrease gut production of B1:

Antibiotics – Aminoglycosides, Cephalosporins, Fluoroquinolones, Quinolones, Macrolides, Penicillins, Sulfonamides, Tetracyclines, Trimethoprin-containing antibiotics, Carbapenems, Monobactams, chloramphenicol, spectinomycin, Streptogramins, vancomycin, Oxalodinones, Lincosamides, Nitrofurans

Increase B1 excretion:

Loop Diuretics – furosemide, bumetanide, ethacrynic acid, torsemide

Decrease B1 levels:

Oral contraceptives – norethindrone, ethynodiol diacetate, norgestrel, norgestimate, ethinyl estradiol, drospirenone, desogestrel, levonorgestrel

Phenytoin, caffeic acid, 5 fluorouracil, insulin, nitrites, polyphenols, pyrithiamine, quercetin, sulfonamides, sulphites, tannic acid, thyroxine.

Alcohol inhibits the absorption of B_1.

TARGET TISSUES

Brain, heart, liver, kidney, peripheral nerves.

Total quantity in the body: 30 mg. Biological half-life in the body: 15 days.

ENZYME SYSTEMS INVOLVED

- Alpha keto glutarate decarboxylases
- Oxidative decarboxylation of pyruvate
- Pyruvate dehydrogenase – required for energy production in the Kreb's cycle
- Thiamine kinase
- Transketolase – required for lipid and fat metabolism, synthesis and maintenance of the myelin sheath
- 2- oxy-glucarate dehydrogenase – required for the synthesis of acetylcholine, GABA and glutarate.

DEFICIENCY SYMPTOMS AS RELATED TO METABOLIC ACTION

Anorexia	due to excess production of pyruvate, fatigue, gastrointestinal complaints, weight loss.
Circulatory and heart complaints	due to reduced energy production.

DEFICIENCY SYMPTOMS AMONGST POPULATION

Non alcoholic psychiatric patients	38%
Geriatric population	33-55%
Alcoholic population	30-80%
AIDS patients	> 23%
Pregnancy	25-30%
Gestational diabetes	>50%

Because there is very little thiamin stored in the body, depletion can occur as quickly as within 14 days.

STRUCTURE OF THIAMINE

Thiamine (Vitamin B₁) + ATP → (TPP-synthetase) → AMP → Thiamine pyrophosphate (TPP)

H⁺ Acidic proton

Thiamine (vitamin B₁) is the dietary precursor to the enzyme cofactor thiamine pyrophosphate **(TPP)** which is critical in a number of metabolic transformations, especially that involving energy production.

Vitamin B$_2$

Riboflavin, flavin adenine dinucleotide (FAD) (active form)

SOURCE

Almonds, asparagus, avocados, barley grass, beans, currants, eggs, milk and dairy products, organ meats, sprouts, wholegrain cereals, yeast, broccoli.

PROCESSING LOSSES

Unstable to alkali and light
Pasteurising milk – 10-20%
Meat and vegetable cooking – 10-20%

FACTORS INCREASING DEMAND

Alcohol, coffee, diabetes, eye fatigue, fevers, heart disease, hyperactivity, jaundice, lactose intolerance, malabsorption, oral contraceptives, smoking, stress, sugar and refined food intake, surgery, thyroid disease, vitamin B$_6$ overload.

FUNCTIONS FACILITATED

Alleviates eye fatigue, activates vitamin B6 and folate, coenzyme in respiratory enzyme system, constituent of flavoproteins i.e. important for Krebs cycle function, growth and development of the foetus, maintenance of the mucosa, epithelial and eye tissues; myelin sheath maintenance, participates in reactions where double bonds are involved, red cell synthesis, redox and respiratory enzymes; reduces oedema or lesion size associated with stroke or traumatic brain injury.

DEFICIENCY MAY CAUSE OR BE ASSOCIATED WITH:

Alopecia, anaemia, angular stomatitis (skin cracking or sores at the corners of the mouth), blood shot eyes, blurred vision, cataracts, cheilosis, conjunctivitis, cracks and sores on lips, cystic anaemia associated with pure red cell hypoplasia of the bone marrow, dermatitis with dryness and greasy scaling, digestive disturbance, enlarged liver, eye fatigue, geographic tongue, glossitis, hyperaesthesia to cold and pain, inflammation of mucus membranes, lesions to eye, magenta tongue, oral, ocular, cutaneous and genital lesions (cutaneous lesions usually affect nasolabial folds, alae nasi, scrotum and labia majora), photophobia, redness to lips, retarded growth of infants, seborrhoeic dermatitis, sensitivity to light, sore tongue, sore throat, vascularization of the cornea, weakness, weight loss.

THERAPEUTIC USES

Acne rosacea, alcoholism, amblyopia, arthritis, blurred vision, cataracts, cheilosis, Crohn's disease, diarrhoea, the elderly, eye irritations, geographic tongue, migraine headaches, neonatal jaundice with phototherapy, photophobia, poor immunity, pregnancy, skin disorders, stress, stroke, traumatic brain injury.

DAILY DOSAGE	
RDA	1.5-2 mg
SR	10-200 mg
Infants	0.6 mg
Children	0.8 mg

For migraine therapy – 400mg/day may be required.

Urinary excretion of <30µg riboflavin/g creatine is associated with clinical signs of riboflavin deficiency. Increased activation of RBC glutathione reductase by B$_2$ is an early sign of deficiency.

EFFECTS OF OVERDOSAGE AND TOXICITY

Essentially non toxic to humans.

TECHNICAL NOTES

SYNERGISTIC NUTRIENTS

Vitamin A, B_1, B_3, B_5, B_6, B_{12}, biotin, chromium, copper, cysteine, folate, glutathione, insulin, iron, magnesium, molybdenum, phosphate, potassium, thyroxine, zinc.

DRUG/NUTRIENT INTERACTIONS

Interfere in the conversion of B_2 to its active form:

Tricyclic antidepressants – amitriptyline, amoxapine, clomipramine, desipramine, doxepin, imipramine, nortriptyline, protryptiline, trimipramine

Interfere with gut synthesis of the vitamin B_2:

Antibiotics – Aminoglycosides, Cephalosporins, Fluoroquinolones, Quinolones, Macrolides, Penicillins, Sulfonamides, Tetracyclines, Trimethoprim-containing antibiotics, Carbapenems, Monobactams, chloramphenicol, spectinomycin, Streptogramins, vancomycin, Oxalodinones, Lincosamides, Nitrofurans

Increase excretion of the vitamin B_2:

Phenothiazines – chlorpromazine, thioridazine, fluphenazine, trifluoperazine, mesoridazine, prochlorperazine, perphenazine, promethazine

Decrease vitamin B_2 absorption:

Cholestyramine, colestipol, cadmium

Decrease B_2 vitamin status:

Oral contraceptives – norethindrone, ethynodiol diacetate, norgestrel, norgestimate, ethinyl estradiol, drospirenone, desogestrel, levonorgestrel

Acetophenazine, Araboflavin, Boric Acid, Doxycycline, Excess Intake of Iron, Copper, Galactoflavin, Isocarboxazid, Manganese, Tranylcypromine, Phenelzine, Probenecid.

NUTRIENT/NUTRIENT INTERACTIONS

Copper, iron and manganese in high doses may interfere with vitamin B_2 status.

TARGET TISSUES

Heart, kidney, liver.

ENZYME SYSTEMS INVOLVED

- Co-enzyme forms are FAD, FMN.
- FAD is involved in most oxidase enzymes – xanthine oxidase, glycine oxidase.
- FMN is involved in the cytochrome enzyme system.
- Glutathione reductase.

DEFICIENCY SYMPTOMS AS RELATED TO METABOLIC ACTION

Glossitis	
seborrhoeic dermatitis	
stomatitis	
cheilosis	
corneal vascularity due to other vitamin deficiencies	as vitamin B_2 activates a number of B vitamins.
Photophobia	synergistic functions with vitamin A.

STRUCTURE VITAMIN B₂/RIBOFLAVIN

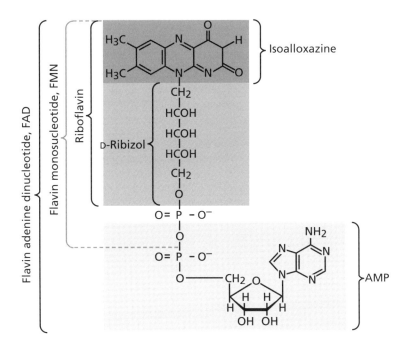

Active form of vitamin B_2 – flavin adenine dinucleotide. (FAD)

Vitamin B₃

Niacin, nicotinic acid, niacinamide
Nicotinamide adenine dinucleotide (NAD)(Active Form) – Coenzyme I,
Nicotinamide adenine dinucleotide phosphate (NADP) – Coenzyme II

SOURCE

Almonds, beef, chicken, eggs, fish, halibut, legumes, mackerel, meat, peanuts, salmon, sardines, sunflower seeds, yeast.

PROCESSING LOSSES

Stable to heating, ethylene oxide used to ripen fruit results in 50% loss in vitamin B_3.

FACTORS INCREASING DEMAND

Alcohol excess, amino acid imbalances, biliary atresia, burns, cirrhosis, coffee excess, diarrhoea, excess intake of sugar, fever, growth spurts, Hartnup's disease, high blood cholesterol, Hodgkin's disease, isoniazid therapy, leukaemia, low protein diets, malabsorption syndrome, malignant carcinoid tumour, maple syrup disease, phenylketonuria, polyuria, refined foods, renal disease, schizophrenia, smoking, ulcerative colitis.

FUNCTIONS FACILITATED

Antineuritic factor, co-factor to enzyme poly (ADP-ribose) polymerase (PARP-1), energy production, hormone and lipid synthesis, lowers blood cholesterol, maintains the respiratory chain enzymes in the mitochondria, metabolism of fats, proteins and carbohydrate; maintains healthy skin, tongue and digestive system; mitochondrial biogenesis, neuroprotective, normalises cancer cell energetics, potentiates anticonvulsant activity, stimulates ATP or energy production, stimulates DNA repair, stimulates tyrosine hydroxylase, stimulates gastric secretion and bile secretion. Nicotinamide modulates or inhibits IL-1B, IL-6, IL-8 and TNF alpha.

NAD functions as an electron carrier for intracellular respiration as well as a cofactor for enzymes involved in the oxidation of fats and carbohydrates, such as: glyceraldehyde 3-phosphate, lactate, pyruvate and alpha-ketoglutarate dehydrogenases. NAD participates in reactions where alcohols are converted to ketones, aldehydes & organic acids.

NADP functions as a hydrogen donor in reductive biosynthesis, such as in fatty acid and steroid synthesis, and like NAD as a cofactor for enzymes, such as in the oxidation of glucose-6- phosphate to ribose 5-phosphate in the pentose phosphate pathway.

DEFICIENCY MAY CAUSE OR BE ASSOCIATED WITH:

Abdominal discomfort and distension, achlorhydria, amenorrhoea, anaemia, anorexia, anxiety, burning mouth, canker sores, Casal's necklace, chronic hypertrophy of skin and chronic atrophic lesions, chronic infections, chronic headaches, confusion, cutaneous lesions, dementia, depression, dermatitis (butter fly rash, hyperkeratotic skin lesions on hands, feet, face and neck [sun exposed regions]), diarrhoea, fatigue, glossitis; gingivitis with tooth loss; Hartnup's disease, headaches, haeme deficiency, hyperpigmentation, indigestion, infertility, inflammation of gut tissues, insomnia; irregular muscular contraction of the tongue; loss of hearing, malignant carcinoid tumour, memory loss, mucosal ulceration, movement disorder – chorea, tremors, rigidity, loss of arm swing; muscular weakness, nausea, night terrors, optic neuritis, Parkinsonism symptoms, pellagra, polyneuropathy, psychosis, restlessness, red tongue, scaly dermatitis, scrotal rashes, scarlet glossitis and stomatitis, schizophrenia, suicidal behaviour; tendency to criminality, violence and social isolation; tremor, tingling fingers, visual and auditory hallucinations, vomiting.

Metabolic disorder – glucose intolerance, diabetes, thyroid disease, Addison's disease, hypopituitarism with diabetes insipudis, disturbed acid/base balance, cachexia, mitochondrial defects.

THERAPEUTIC USES

Adeno-carcinoma of the stomach, alcoholism, anxiety, arthritis, atherosclerosis, burns, cancer, cholera patients, coronary artery disease, cramps, depression, diabetes, Hartnup's disease, high blood cholesterol, Hodgkin's disease, hypertension, hypertriglyceremia, mitochondrial disease, neuritis, night terrors, optic neuritis, pellagra, poor circulation, polyneuropathy, psychosis, protein deficiency and imbalances, schizophrenia, smoking withdrawal, tooth growth, traumatic brain injury, UV induced skin tumours.

NAD – Alzheimer's disease, anxiety, canker sores, chronic fatigue, dementia, depression, Huntington's disease, infection, Parkinson's disease, poor memory, mitochondrial pathology.

DAILY DOSAGE	
RDA	15-20 mg
SR	100-3000 mg
SR for Activated B₃ (NAD)	5-10 mg/day
Infants	5-6 mg
Children (1-3 yrs)	9-13 mg

EFFECTS OF OVERDOSAGE AND TOXICITY

Niacin or nicotinic acid has limited toxicity. Most adverse effects are dose related and generally subside with a reduction in dose or the cessation of treatment.

Dosage > 1-4 g/day
Acute Toxicity
flushing, itching of the skin, nausea, vomiting, gastrointestinal disturbances, diarrhoea. Increase in pulse and respiration rate. Taking aspirin or non-steroidal anti-inflammatory drugs such as: ibuprofen, naproxen or indomethacin, can reduce the flushing.

Chronic Toxicity
(generally intakes of 3,000 mg/day or more) for long periods of time:

jaundice, hyperglycemia, abdominal pain, elevated serum bilirubin, alkaline phosphatase and aminotransferase, fatty liver, hyperuremia.

Sustained release preparations are reported to be more hepatotoxic than the crystalline form.

Niacinamide: >2g:
Inhibits PARP-1 and this may cause genomic instability.

Nicotinamide is metabolised to methylnicotinamide which can increase the need for methyl groups. Methionine or SAMe may need to be provided if large doses of niacin or nicotinamide are taken.

TECHNICAL NOTES

SYNERGISTIC NUTRIENTS

Vitamin B_1, B_2, B_6, B_{12}, C, chromium, zinc, potassium, manganese, chromium, phosphorus, copper, folic acid, iron, leucine, magnesium, methionine, SAMe, molybdenum, potassium, selenium, tryptophan.

DRUG/NUTRIENT INTERACTIONS

Decrease gut synthesis of vitamin B$_3$:
Antibiotics – Aminoglycosides, Cephalosporins, Fluoroquinolones, Quinolones, Macrolides, Penicillins, Sulfonamides, Tetracyclines, Trimethoprin-containing antibiotics, Carbapenems, Monobactams, chloramphenicol, spectinomycin, Streptogramins, vancomycin, Oxalodinones, Lincosamides, Nitrofurans

Reduce body levels of vitamin B$_3$:
Isoniazid, 5-Fluoronicotinic Acid, Bleomycin, Isonicotinic Acid, Metronidazole, Thalidomide.

Vitamin B$_3$ increases drug toxicity by interfering with drug metabolism
Anticonvulsants – primidone, carbamazepine

TARGET TISSUES

Gastrointestinal tract, heart, kidney, liver, muscle, skin, spinal cord.

ENZYME SYSTEMS INVOLVED

- Co-enzyme forms – NAD, NADP.
- Involved in more than fifty biochemical reactions.
- Activates dehydrogenases, oxidases, mixed function oxidases.
- Participates in reactions where alcohols are converted to ketones, aldehydes and organic acids.

DEFICIENCY SYMPTOMS AS RELATED TO METABOLIC ACTION	
Dermatitis, itching skin, pigmentation, tongue lesions	other vitamins involved, particularly B$_2$.
Irritability, mental disturbances	synergism with B$_1$.
Retarded growth	general synergism of all vitamins.

STRUCTURE VITAMIN B3

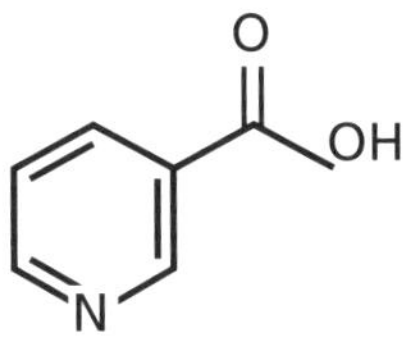

nicotinic acid
(niacin)

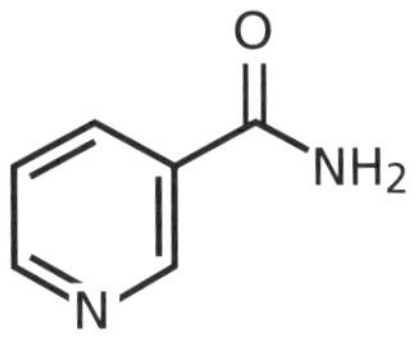

nicotinamide
(niacinamide)

STRUCTURE OF ACTIVE FORM OF VITAMIN B3 – NICOTINAMIDE ADENINE DINUCLEOTIDE (NAD AND NADP)

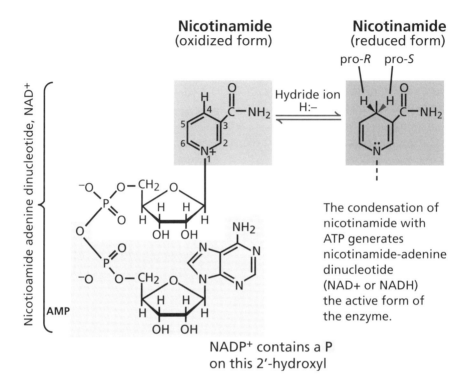

Nicotinamide (oxidized form)

Nicotinamide (reduced form)

pro-*R*   pro-*S*

Hydride ion H:−

Nicotioamide adenine dinucleotide, NAD⁺

AMP

NADP⁺ contains a P on this 2'-hydroxyl

The condensation of nicotinamide with ATP generates nicotinamide-adenine dinucleotide (NAD+ or NADH) the active form of the enzyme.

The condensation of nicotinamide with ATP generates nicotinamide-adenine dinucleotide (NAD+ or NADH), the active form of the enzyme.

Vitamin B₅

Pantothenic Acid

SOURCE

Avocado, baker's yeast, beans, brains, blue vein cheese, egg yolk, green vegetables, heart, kidney, lentils, liver, lobsters, milk, mushrooms, oranges, peas, royal jelly, sweet potatoes, wholegrain cereals.

PROCESSING LOSSES

Unstable to heat, alkali and acid

Considerable loss in milling of grains

Frozen vegetables 50%, cooking up to 44%, canning 75%

FACTORS INCREASING DEMAND

Ageing, arthritis, depression, elevated urinary hippuric acid, fluid retention, high intakes of alcohol and coffee, mercury exposure, pregnancy, streptomycin toxicity, stress, weakness.

FUNCTIONS FACILITATED

Involved in the synthesis of acetylcholine, antibody production, carries activated acetyl group, cholesterol, cortisone, decreases lactic acid accumulation in tissues, improves body's resistance to stress, precursor to cysteic acid, fibroblast multiplication, steroid hormone production, strengthens the immune system, ketones, lipid metabolism, constituent of coenzyme A, protein metabolism, reduces arthritic pain, maintains normal uric acids levels, sphingosine.

DEFICIENCY MAY CAUSE OR BE ASSOCIATED WITH:

Abdominal pains, alopecia, anaemia, arthritis, burning feet, convulsions, coordination impairment, depression, dermatitis, digestive and cardiovascular disorders, fatigue, fertility problems, hyper-irritability, hypotension, infections, insomnia, itching, kidney stones, malaise, muscle spasms or cramps, nervousness, paraesthesia, poor immunity, restlessness, sleep disturbances, tenderness of heels, vomiting.

THERAPEUTIC USES

Adrenal stress, alcoholism, allergies, arthritis, asthma, autonomic dysfunction, burning feet syndrome, constipation, chronic bronchitis, coordination impairment, cramps, decreased serum potassium, demyelination, detoxification of benzoic acid, diabetes, eczema, episodic nocturnal motor hyperfunction, failure of adrenocorticotropin to induce eosinopenia, fluid retention, growth retardation, hair dryness, hair loss, impaired coordination, infections, insomnia, itching, liver disease, lowered plasma cholesterol, nervousness, oral mucosa ulcer, osteoarthritis, personality changes, panic attacks, polyneuritis, poor immunity, radium treatment, rheumatoid arthritis, rhinitis, skin disease, ulcerative colitis, varicose ulcers, wound healing.

DAILY DOSAGE	
RDA	5-10 mg
SR	20-500 mg

RDA by age:	
0-0.5 yrs	2 mg
0.5-3 yrs	3 mg
4-6 yrs	3-4 mg
7-10 yrs	4-5 mg
11 yrs	4-7 mg

EFFECTS OF OVERDOSAGE AND TOXICITY

Essentially non-toxic in humans.

Dosage > 10 gm

increase in histamine and sensitivity in joints and possibly diarrhoea.

TECHNICAL NOTES

SYNERGISTIC NUTRIENTS

Vitamin B_1, B_2, B_3, B_{12}, C, biotin, chromium, cysteine, folate, glycine, methionine, phosphate, sodium, potassium, zinc.

DRUG/NUTRIENT INTERACTIONS

Decrease Vitamin B5 status:

Salicylates – aspirin, choline salicylate, sodium salicylate, magnesium salicylate, salsalate, diflunisal, sodium thiosalicylate

Chemotherapeutics, High Copper Intake, Oral Contraceptives, Para-Aminosalicylic Acid, Streptomycin, Sulfonamide.

TARGET TISSUES

All tissues; particularly brain, heart, kidney, liver.

ENZYME SYSTEM INVOLVED

- Coenzyme form – CoA and phospho-pantetheine.
- Activates dehydrogenases, esterases, hydrases, isomerases, synthetases, transacylases, transferases.
- Carries activated acetyl groups.

DEFICIENCY SYMPTOMS AS RELATED TO METABOLIC ACTION

Cardiovascular disorders	disturbances of fat and carbohydrate metabolism due to liver degeneration.
Digestive disorders	decreased bile acid production due to decreased sterol production, atrophy of intestinal mucosa.
Neuromotor disturbance	decreased synthesis of phospholipid and acetylcholine.

STRUCTURE FOR PANTOTHENIC ACID

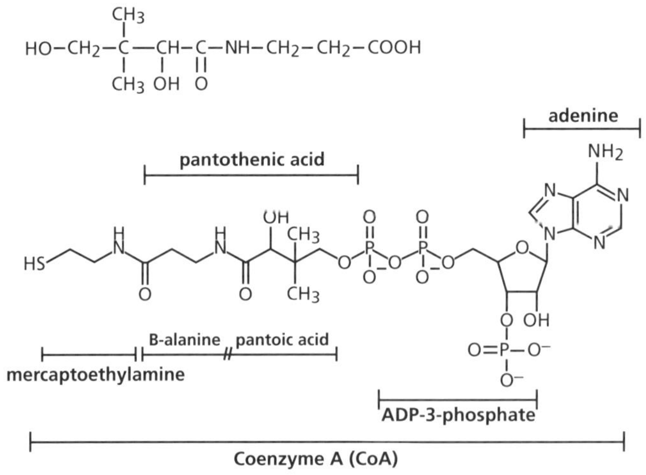

Pantothenic is a precursor to Coenzyme A. The structure consists of beta-alanine in amide linkage with pantoic acid; the key functional group is the -SH group to which fatty acids are attached by thio-ester linkage during the process of fatty acid synthesis.

Vitamin B$_6$

Pyridoxine, Co-decarboxylase Hydrochloride, Pyridoxal-5-phosphate [P-5-P] (active form) and Pyridoxamine phosphate

SOURCE

Avocado, bananas, brewer's yeast, carrot, cereal, chicken, egg yolk, ham, legumes, lentils, mackerel, oatmeal, offal, peanuts, salmon, tuna, sunflower seeds, walnuts.

PROCESSING LOSSES

Unstable to light.

Milling flour – 75%, cooking – 30-45%.

FACTORS INCREASING DEMAND

Ageing, abdominal surgery, alcoholism, cancer (breast, cervical, pancreatic), chemical sensitivity, coeliac disease, diabetes, excessive intakes of coffee, tea, alcohol, cigarettes, and protein; fever or febrile states, gyrate atrophy, helps the release of glucose from glycogen, homocystinuria, hypertension, isoniazid ingestion, kidney stones, lactation, methionine loading, oral contraceptives, pregnancy, radium therapy, regulates steroid hormone action, schizophrenics, uraemic patients, xanthurenic aciduria, uremia.

Factors Increasing Demand For P-5-P

Asthma, hypertension, methionine loading, pancreatic and cervical cancer.

FUNCTIONS FACILITATED

Carbohydrate metabolism, cofactor in the synthesis of vitamin B$_3$, decreases platelet aggregation (by inhibiting glycoprotein IIb), decreases AGE formation, hormone synthesis, involved in synthesis of essential fatty acid metabolites (prostaglandins), increases aldose reductase activity, improves oxygenation of tissues, lipid metabolism, neurotransmitter synthesis (serotonin, dopamine, noradrenaline, GABA, his-tamine), protein metabolism, reduces androgenic and oestrogenic transcription response, supports optimum nervous system function.

Pyridoxal-5-phosphate:

Inhibits angiogenesis, down-regulates the activity of RNA polymerase, reverses transcriptase and DNA polymerase; inhibits glycoprotein IIb – a protein that is involved in platelet aggregation, modulator of steroid and albumin gene expression.

DEFICIENCY MAY CAUSE OR BE ASSOCIATED WITH:

Abdominal distress, abnormal electro encephalogram, acne, anaemia – lymphopenia with eosinophilia, anorexia, arteriosclerosis, ascending sensory polyneuropathy, cheilosis, conjunctivitis, confusion, convulsions, depression, dermatitis, facial oiliness, fatigue, glossitis, hyperirritability, hypochromic microcytic anaemia, increased excretion of xanthurenic acid, increased susceptibility to virus induced tumour growth, increased tissue sensitivity to steroid hormone stimulation, insomnia, kidney stones, lethargy, low blood sugar, lymphopenia, nausea, neuronal dysfunction, poor coordination in walking, poor immunity, pre-menstrual fluid retention, sensorimotor neuropathy, skin lesions, seizures, sleepiness, sleep walking, vomiting, weakness, weight loss.

THERAPEUTIC USES

Allergy, anaemia, anxiety, arthritis, asthma, atherosclerosis, athletic performance, autism, breast cancer, carpal tunnel syndrome, chemically sensitive individuals, coeliac disease, Crohn's disease, cyclosporine therapy, dysmenorrhoea, the elderly, epilepsy, glossitis, Gyrate atrophy of the retina and choroid, hand numbness, hereditary sideroblastic anemia, homocystinuria, hypoglycaemia, hypoxia; improves survival time in patients with cervical carcinoma, stage P endometrial carcinoma, stage P bladder cancer and breast cancer; inborn errors of metabolism, infertility, liver disease, leg cramps, mental retardation, memory deficits, muscular disorder, nausea of pregnancy, Parkinson's disease, premenstrual fluid retention, radiation sickness, schizophrenia, seizures in new born, sleep walking, stiffness of the hands, stress, sun sensitivity, uraemic patients.

Therapeutic uses of P-5-P
Arrhythmias, coronary artery disease, cervical and pancreatic cancer, homocystinuria, hypertension, hyperglycaemia, gyrate atrophy, myocardial infarction.

DAILY DOSAGE	
RDA	1.6-2.6 mg
SR	10-150 mg
P-5-P supplementary range	10-50mg

RDA by age:	
0-0.5 yrs	0.3 mg
0.5-1 yrs	0.6 mg
1-3 yrs	1.0 mg
4-6 yrs	1.1 mg
7-10 yrs	1.4 mg
11-14 yrs	4-7 mg
Male Adults	2.0 mg
Female Adults	1.6 mg
Lactation	2.0 mg

EFFECTS OF OVERDOSAGE AND TOXICITY

Limited toxicity in humans. May cause skin eruptions or worsening of acne vulgaris.

Dosages > 500mg
Coordination problems, tonic convulsions, (over 3 years) peripheral neuropathy, progressive sensory ataxia, loss of vibratory sense. Inhibits myelin synthesis.

Neuropathy due to toxicity occurs 1 month to 3 years after the individual starts excessive consumption. Toxicity symptoms are reversed on discontinuation.

TECHNICAL NOTES

SYNERGISTIC NUTRIENTS
Vitamin B_1, B_2, B_3, B_5, B_{12}, C, E, biotin, chromium, copper, folate, magnesium, potassium, phosphate, selenium, sodium, zinc.

DRUG/NUTRIENT INTERACTIONS

Vitamin B_6 may increase the breakdown of levodopa in the body, possibly altering the effectiveness of this medication.

Decrease gut synthesis of vitamin B_6:
  Antibiotics – Aminoglycosides, Cephalosporins, Fluoroquinolones, Quinolones, Macrolides, Penicillins, Sulfonamides, Tetracyclines, Trimethoprin-containing antibiotics, Carbapenems, Monobactams, chloramphenicol, spectinomycin, Streptogramins, vancomycin, Oxalodinones, Lincosamides, Nitrofurans

Increase excretion of vitamin B_6:
  Loop diuretics – furosemide, bumetanide, ethacrynic acid, torsemide
  Thiazide diuretics

Reduce Vitamin B$_6$ status:

Estrogen and estrogen-like medications – conjugated estrogens, estradiol, estrone, esterified estrogens, estropipate, ethinyl estradiol, raloxifene, transdermal estradiol, vaginal estrogens.

Hydralazine, Isoniazid, Amino-Oxyacetic Acid, Amphetamine, Chlorpromazine, Cycloserine, Ethionamide, Furfural, Hydrazide, Hydrazine, Hydroxylamine, Insulin, Marijuana, Penicillamine, Pyrazinamide, Reserpine, Semicarbazide, Steroids Thiosemicarbazone.

Interupt Vitamin B$_6$ metabolism:
Penicillamine, Theophylline

Vitamin B$_6$ depleting medications (influence melatonin synthesis):

Conjugated estrogens, estradiol, estrone, esterified estrogens, estropipate, ethinyl estradiol, progesterone, medroxyprogesterone, hydroxyprogesterone, norethindrone, ethynodiol diacetate, norgestrel, norgestimate, drospirenone, desogestrel, levonorgestrel, antibiotics, nitroglycerin (various dosage forms), isosorbide mononitrate, isosorbide dinitrate, amyl nitrate, isoxsuprine, hydralazine, minoxidil, papaverine, tolazoline, epoprostenol, ethaverine, nesiritide, bosentan, furosemide, bumetanide, ethacrynic acid, torsemide, theophylline, isoniazid, penicillamine, phenelzine.

Amino-oxyacetic acid, amphetamine, chlorpromazine, cycloserine, ethionamide, furfural, hydrazide, hydrazine, hydroxylamine, insulin, marijuana, penicillamine, pyrazinamide, reserpine, semicarbazide, steroids, thiosemicarbazone.

TARGET TISSUES

Liver, lymph nodes, muscle tissue, nervous tissue.

ENZYME SYSTEMS INVOLVED

Involved in 120 different enzyme systems – mainly in carboxylation and transamination reactions.

- Co-enzyme forms – Co decarboxylase (pyridoxal-5-phospate) pyridoxamine phosphate.
- Activates – amino acid decarboxylases, dehydrases (porphyrin synthesis phosphorylases), desulfhydrases (cysteine), oxidases (diamine), phenylalanine metabolism, transaminases (glutamic, aspartic), tryptophan and tyrosine metabolism.

DEFICIENCY SYMPTOMS AS RELATED TO METABOLIC FUNCTION	
Skin lesions	Synergism of B$_6$ with B$_2$ and B$_3$ for skin maintenance.
Convulsion	Involved in the production of: neurotransmitters, dopamine, serotonin, noradrenaline, GABA.
Xanthurenic acid excretion	B$_6$ required for kynureninase enzyme.
Anaemia	Synergism of B$_6$ with B$_{12}$ for red blood cell formation.

STRUCTURES VITAMIN B$_6$

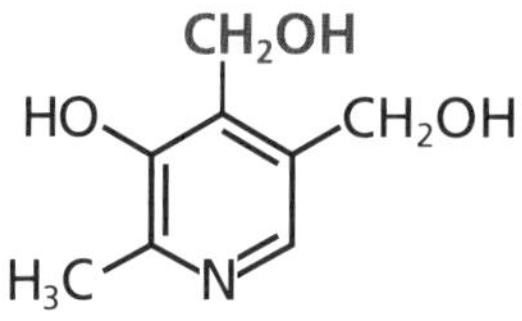

Pyridoxine

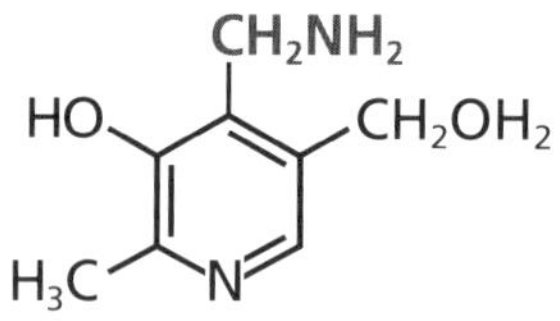

Pyridoxamine

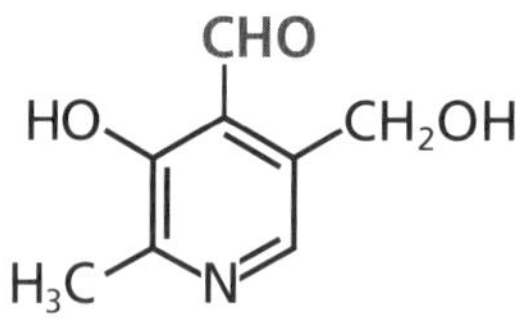

Pyridoxal

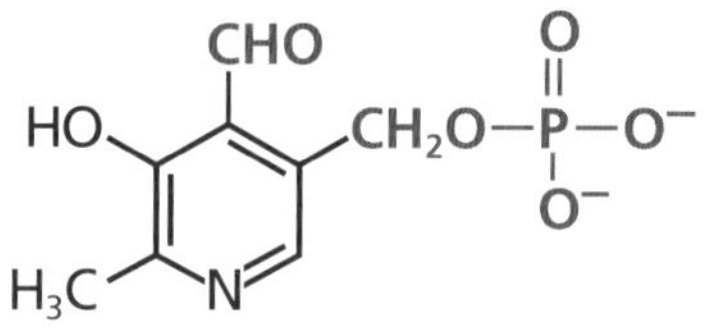

Pyridoxal phosphate

The active form of vitamin B$_6$ is pyridoxal-5-phosphate. It plays a role in metabolising glycine, tryptophan, tyrosine, serotonin, glutamate and sulphur amino acids.

Vitamin B$_{12}$

Cobalamin, Cyanocobalamin, Methylcobalamin, adenosyl-cobalamin

SOURCE

Bacterial synthesis occurs in the gut. Found in: brain, clams, egg yolk, herring, kidney, liver, liver wurst, meat, milk, oysters, salmon, sardines, Swiss cheese.

PROCESSING LOSSES

Unstable to heat, light, alkali, and acid Losses range from 10-90%

FACTORS INCREASING DEMAND

Ageing, anaemia, anorexia, bacterial overgrowth in the gut, blind loop surgery, cancer, chemical sensitivity, chronic fatigue syndrome, chronic pancreatitis, Crohn's disease, coeliac disease, diabetes, diverticulitis, excessive intakes of alcohol and tobacco, fibromyalgia, gastrectomy, gastric mucosal atrophy, hyperthyroidism, inflammation, inflammatory bowel disease, inflammatory conditions, infections-tape worm, tropical sprue, lactation, laxative abuse, liver and kidney disease, mature onset schizophrenia, multiple sclerosis, osteoarthritis, pancreatic insufficiency, pregnancy, sprue, short bowel syndrome, tape worm infestations, thyrotoxicosis, ulcerative colitis, vegetarianism.

FUNCTIONS FACILITATED

Biosynthesis of nucleic acids, DNA, protein and blood cells; maintenance of normal bone marrow, gut mucosa, epithelial cells and body lipids; increases synthesis of methionine synthetase, maintenance of growth, maintenance of differentiation, proliferation and metabolic status of cells, metabolism of fat, protein and carbohydrate; methyl group transfer or methylation reactions, modulates TNF expression, myelination of nerve and brain fibres. Quenches nitric oxide (NO) and is a source of cobalt.

Methylcobalamin is essential for folate metabolism and the formation of choline containing phospholipids. The most active form of B$_{12}$, required for the methylation cycle, protects cortical neurons against NMDA glutamate receptor activity, regulates circadian rhythms, improves concentration, alertness and sleep quality.

Adenosylcobalamin (dibencozide) is required for the formation of succinyl coenzyme A, which is involved in the formation of neural lipids. It is essential for energy metabolism, required for normal myelin sheath production and nucleoprotein production. Deficiency gives rise to nerve and spinal cord degeneration.

Cyanocobalamin a synthetic form of vitamin B$_{12}$ of low biological activity, converted in the liver to a more active form.

Hydroxycobalamin is a potent NO scavenger, detoxifies cyanide, the smokers and cassava eaters choice of B$_{12}$. Cytoprotective and helps recycle methioine.

DEFICIENCY MAY CAUSE OR BE ASSOCIATED WITH:

AIDS, achlorhydria, agitation, anaemia, apathy, ataxia, attention deficit disorder, bladder or bowel incontinence, brown discolouration of joints, chromosome breaks, chronic inflammation, cofactor in the production of succinyl-Co A, concentration difficulties, cranial artery dissection, decreased blood tissue lipids, dementia, demyelination of spinal chord, brain, optic and peripheral nerves; depression, diminished lower limb vibratory sense, dizziness, fatigue, heart pain, increased excretion of methylmalonic acid, inflammation of tongue, impaired vibration and joint position sense, impairs folate metabolism, impairs folate metabolism & hence DNA synthesis, irritability, laboured breathing, leukopenia, memory loss, mood swings, negativism, neurological lesions, neutrophil hypersegmentation, numbness, optic neuropathy, organic brain syndrome, pale smooth tongue, paranoia, parasthesia, peripheral neuropathy, poor appetite, psychosis, restlessness, retarded growth, schizophrenia, spinal lesions, sprue, symmetrical numbness of hands and feet, temper outbursts, tingling, violence, weakness, weight loss.

THERAPEUTIC USES

Achlorhydria, acne vulgaris, alcoholism, allergy, amblyopia, anaemia (megoblastic), aphthous stomatitis, arthritis, attention deficit, atrophic gastritis, bronchial asthma, bladder or bowel incontinence, bursitis, cardiovascular disease, calcium bone spurs, chemically sensitive individuals, chromosome breaks, chronic inflammation, chronic inflammatory condition, coeliac disease, cognitive impairment, confusion, Crohn's disease, dementia, depression, diabetes mellitus, functional psychosis, herpes zoster (shingles), high B_{12} levels, homocystinuria, ileitis, infection, insomnia, memory loss, metabisulfite sensitivity, multiple sclerosis, nursing mothers, pancreatic insufficiency, parasthesia, peripheral neuropathy, pernicious anaemia, post partum depression, presentation of neural tube defects, restlessness, shingles, senile dementia, sepsis, systemic inflammatory response syndrome, sepsis, septic traumatic shock, systemic inflammatory response syndrome

(SIRS), trauma, ulcerative colitis, vegetarians, violent behaviour, Zollinger-Ellison syndrome.

DAILY DOSAGE	
RDA	2-50 µg
SR	300-8000 µg
RDA by age:	
0-0.5 yrs	0.3 µg
0.5-1 yrs	0.5 µg
1-6 yrs	1.0 µg
7-10 yrs	1.4 µg
Adults	2.0 µg
Pregnancy & Lactation	2.6 µg

EFFECTS OF OVERDOSAGE AND TOXICITY
General lack of toxicity. Polycythemia reported.

TECHNICAL NOTES

SYNERGISTIC NUTRIENTS

Vitamin A, B_1, B_2, B_5, B_6, C, E, biotin, calcium, cobalt, copper, folate, iron, methionine, N-acetyl cysteine, omega -3 fatty acids, phosphate, selenium.

DRUG/NUTRIENT INTERACTIONS
Decrease body levels of vitamin B_{12}: **Oral contraceptives** – norethindrone, ethynodiol diacetate, norgestrel, norgestimate, ethinyl estradiol, drospirenone, desogestrel, levonorgestrel.
Antivirals Nucleoside Reverse Transcriptase Inhibitors – zidovudine (azidothymidine; AZT; compound S), didanosine (ddI; dideoxyinosine), lamivudine (3TC), stavudine (d4T), zalcitabine (ddC; dideoxycytidine), abacavir sulfate.

Reduce gut synthesis of the vitamin:
Antibiotics – Aminoglycosides, Cephalosporins, Fluoroquinolones, Quinolones, Macrolides, Penicillins, Sulfonamides, Tetracyclines, Trimethoprin-containing antibiotics, Carbapenems, Monobactams, chloramphenicol, spectinomycin, Streptogramins, vancomycin, Oxalodinones, Lincosamides, Nitrofurans.

Decrease B$_{12}$ absorption:
Biguanides – metformin, phenformin
Bile acid sequestrants – cholestyramine, colestipol, colesevelam
H-2 receptor antagonists – cimetidine, famotidine, nizatidine, ranitidine
Proton pump inhibitors – lansoprazole, omeprazole, rabeprazole, pantoprazole, esomeprazole
Potassium chloride, sustained/ controlled release medications – potassium chloride

Clofibrate, Colchicine, Chlor-colchicine, Fenofibrate, Phenytoin, Calcium carbonate.

Reduces vitamin B$_{12}$ status:
Aminosalicylic Acid, Anilide, Cellulose, Cephalosporin, Dilantin, Ethanol, Ethylamide, Methyl-Amide, Pectin, Para-Aminosalicylic Acid, Pteridine, Slow Release Potassium Iodide.

TARGET TISSUE

Bones, central nervous system, heart, kidney, muscle, skin. Stomach secretes intrinsic factor that binds B$_{12}$ and mediates its absorption by receptor sites in the ileum.

- Co-enzyme forms – adenyl cobalamide coenzyme (adenyl nucleoside); 5, 6, dimethyl-benzimidazolyl-cobamide coenzyme.
- Activates mutases (glutamic, methylmalonyl).
- Dehydrases (diol, glycerol, ethanolamine).
- Transmethylases (B$_{12}$ enzyme).

Reductases (ribonucleotide acetate synthesis enzymes).

DEFICIENCY SYMPTOMS AS RELATED TO METABOLIC ACTION	
Disturbed sugar metabolism	methylmalonic acid mutase requires vitamin B$_{12}$.
Gut changes	decreased cell division of gastric mucosa.
Leukopenia	decreased DNA synthesis in stem cells.
Megaloblastic anaemia	decreased DNA synthesis with folate.
Spinal chord changes	decreased RNA synthesis.

BLOOD LEVELS

Normal Range: 500-1300µg/l

STRUCTURE OF VITAMIN B₁₂/CYANOCOBALAMINE

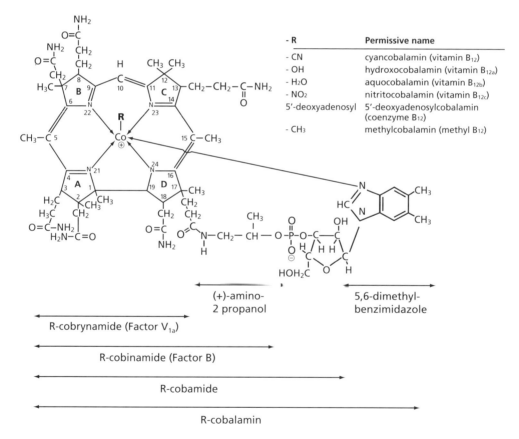

- R	Permissive name
- CN	cyancobalamin (vitamin B_{12})
- OH	hydroxocobalamin (vitamin B_{12a})
- H_2O	aquocobalamin (vitamin B_{12b})
- NO_2	nitritocobalamin (vitamin B_{12c})
5'-deoxyadenosyl	5'-deoxyadenosylcobalamin (coenzyme B_{12})
- CH_3	methylcobalamin (methyl B_{12})

(+)-amino-2 propanol

5,6-dimethyl-benzimidazole

R-cobrynamide (Factor V₁ₐ)

R-cobinamide (Factor B)

R-cobamide

R-cobalamin

Beta-carotene

Beta-carotene is part of a large family of compounds known as Carotenoids

SOURCE
Broccoli, carrots, yellow and greenish yellow vegetables, crude palm oil, papaya, red peppers, spinach, sweet potatoes, tomatoes.

PROCESSING LOSSES
Unstable to heat and light

FACTORS INCREASING DEMAND
Ageing, cystic fibrosis, pesticide exposure, smoking.

FUNCTIONS FACILITATED
Activation of macrophages and lymphocytes, antioxidant, decreases T suppressor activity, increases LDL resistance to oxidation, increases HDL levels, increases interferon activity, increases number of natural killer cells, inhibitor of ornithine decarboxylase, inhibits plaque cell formation, precursor of vitamin A, protects skin against sunburn, reduces the size of cancers, prevents oxidation damage to DNA, RNA, cell proteins and membranes; singlet oxygen quencher.

Protects mucous membranes of the mouth, nose, throat and lungs.

DEFICIENCY MAY CAUSE OR BE ASSOCIATED WITH:
Atrophic gastritis, cancer, cataracts, LDL oxidation.

THERAPEUTIC USES
Air pollution exposure, atherosclerosis, cancer, cardiovascular disease, cataract prevention, chemotherapy, cystic fibrosis, degenerative diseases, erythropoietic protoporphyria, high LDL levels, night blindness, HIV infections, macular degeneration, oral cancers, oral leucoplakia; photosensitivity, pesticide exposure, radiation, smokers, surgery.

DAILY DOSAGE	
RDA	5-8 mg
SR	10-40 mg

Conversion to vitamin A (6μg Beta-carotene = 1mg retinol or 3mg = 5000IU of vitamin A).

Less than 50% of beta-carotene is converted to vitamin A.

Supplementation > 15mg must be given with antioxidant vitamin supplementation i.e. with vitamin E, selenium, Co enzyme Q_{10}.

EFFECTS OF OVERDOSAGE > 60mg
Hypercarotenaemia is associated with orange colouration of the skin and with reversible leukopenia, enlarged liver, low blood pressure, weakness, weight loss.
Doses as low as 20mg daily have been associated with increased risk of lung and prostate cancer in adults who smoke.
Plasma concentration of beta-carotene below 0.25 μmole/L, has also been associated with an increased risk of cancer. Eating disorders, kidney disorders, and liver diseases, may cause high blood levels of beta-carotene.

TECHNICAL NOTES

SYNERGISTIC NUTRIENTS

Vitamin A, E, Co enzyme Q_{10}, lipoic acid, selenium.

DRUG/NUTRIENT INTERACTIONS

Cholestyramine, Probucol (reduces plasma levels of lycopene).

Decrease Absorption:
  Bile acid sequestrants –
  cholestyramine, colestipol, colesevelam
  Proton pumps inhibitors –
  lansoprazole, omeprazole, rabeprazole, pantoprazole, esomeprazole.
  Colchicine, mineral oil, Neomycin

Decreases body levels:
  Orlistat

Fish oil increases beta-carotene requirement.

Thyroxine increases conversion of beta-carotene to vitamin A.

Reduces the side effects of:
Beta-methoxypsoralen, quinidine.

TARGET TISSUES

Fatty tissues, liver.

Absorption can be poor. Better absorbed with fatty meals

ENZYME SYSTEMS INVOLVED

• Inhibits ornithine decarboxylase.
• Singlet oxygen quencher.

DEFICIENCY SYMPTOMS AS RELATED TO METABOLIC ACTION

Lipid antioxidant

TECHNICAL NOTES

Carotenes refer to carotenoids that contain only carbon and hydrogen e.g. beta-carotene, alpha carotene, and lycopene.

Beta-carotene and alpha carotene are responsible for the orange colour of carrots.

Lycopene – Responsible for the red colour of tomatoes. Associated with decreased risk of cancer (prostate, breast, lung, endometrium) and cardiovascular diseases; reduces LDL cholesterol; singlet oxygen quencher; up-regulates cell gap junction communication by increasing connexion 43 activity; works synergistically with vitamin D and lutein.

Antioxidant ranking: lycopene > α-tocopherol > α-carotene > ß-cryptoxanthin > zeaxanthin=ß-carotene > lutein.

Xanthophylls – are compounds which contain hydroxyl groups e.g. lutein, zeaxanthin, beta cryptoxanthin or keto groups e.g. canthaxanthin, or both e.g. astaxanthin.

Astaxanthin – Imparts red or pink colour to salmon and lobsters. Antioxidant effective against singlet oxygen, superoxide anion radical, hydrogen peroxide and peroxy radical Inhibited liver tumorigenesis.

Carotenoids are better absorbed in foods that are cooked or steamed.

CAROTENOID BIOLOGICAL EFFECTS

Function	Accessory pigments in photosynthesis, protection against photosensitization, provitamin A.
Actions	Antioxidant, immune enhancement, inhibition of mutagenesis, chemoprevention of carcinogenesis; inhibition of premalignant lesions, screening pigment

30   CHAPTER 1 – Vitamins

Actions (cont)	in fovea (eye), prevents the oxidation of LDL, decreases the risk of macular degeneration and cataracts; decreases risk of some cancers (laryngeal, gastric, cervical cancer, cervical dysplasia and invasive bladder cancer); reduces cardiovascular disease, decreases DNA damage
	in white blood cells; singlet oxygen scavenging, excess energy dissipation and structure stabilization.

THERAPEUTIC USES OF LYCOPENE

Breast, stomach and prostatic cancer, reduces PSA, reduces the risks associated with smoking.

DOSAGE	
RDI	30-40 mg
SR	40-100 mg

STRUCTURE OF CAROTENOIDS

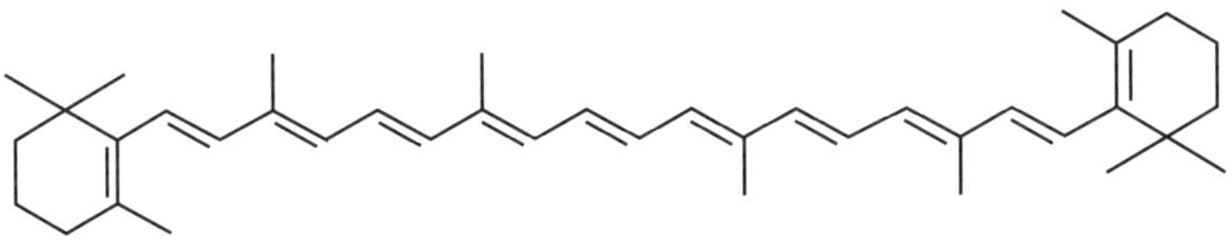

all trans beta carotene

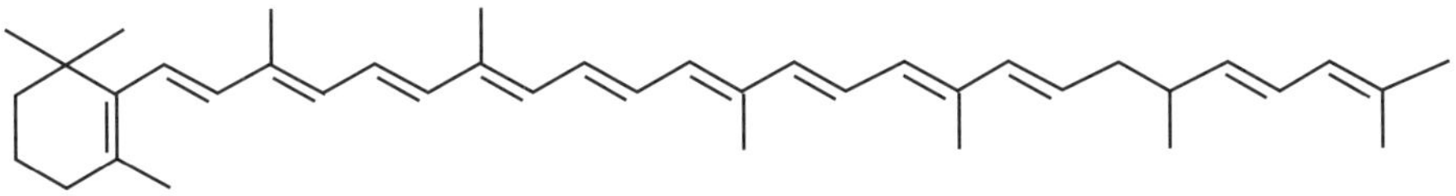

gamma carotene

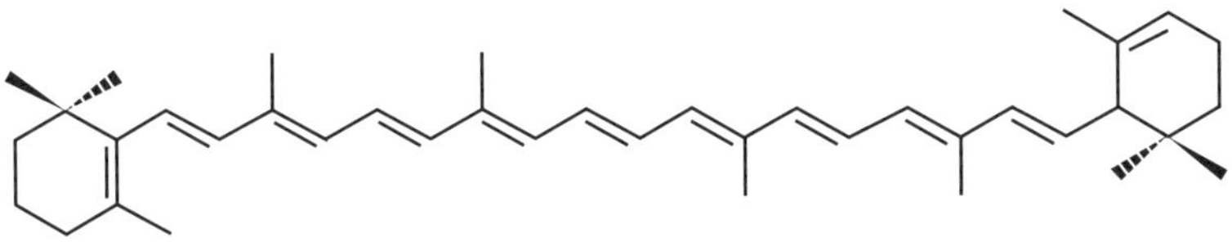

all trans-alpha-carotene

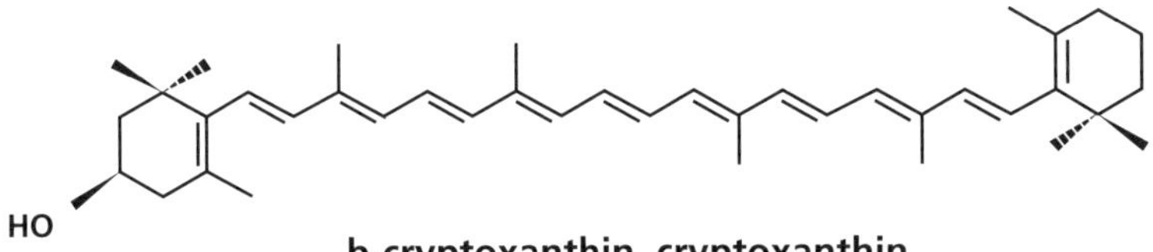

b-cryptoxanthin, cryptoxanthin

STRUCTURE OF ZEAXANTHIN

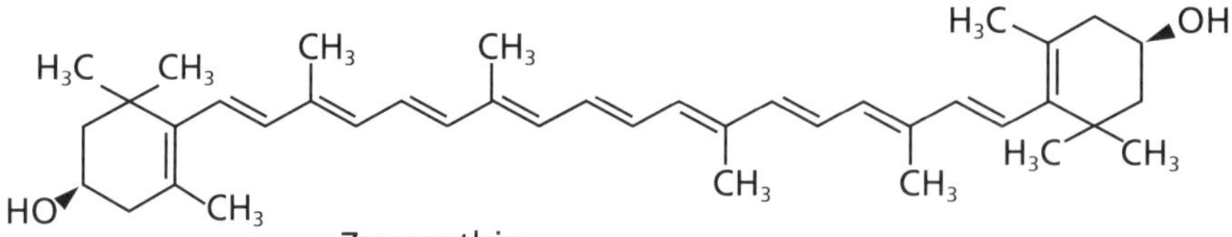

Zeaxanthin

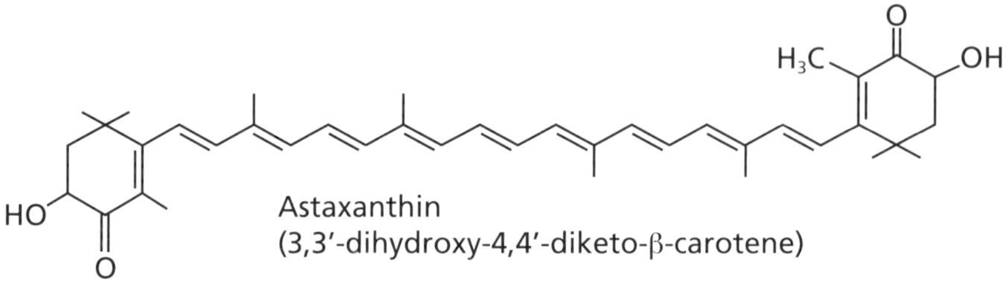

Astaxanthin
(3,3'-dihydroxy-4,4'-diketo-β-carotene)

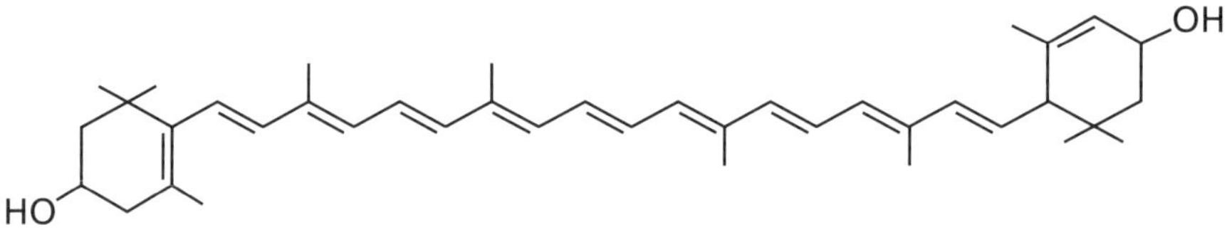

Lutein

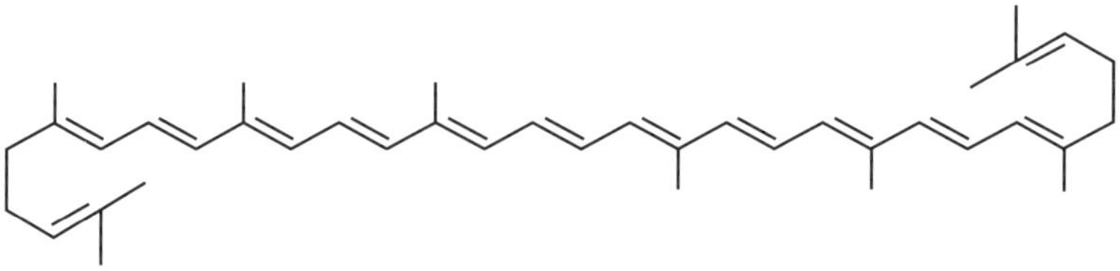

Lycopene
Molecular Weight: 536.89
Molecular Formula: $C_{40}H_{56}$

Bioflavonoids

Citrin, Hesperidin, Rutin, Quercetin. See also – Isoflavones

SOURCE

Apricots, apples, black currants, blue and red berries, buckwheat, cherries, citrus fruit, garlic, green growing shoots of all plants, lemons, olives, onions, red wine, rose hips, skins of fruits, vegetables and soy products.

PROCESSING LOSSES

Some loss during cooking and processing

FACTORS INCREASING DEMAND

Allergies, asthma, high blood pressure, burns, capillary fragility, cataracts, depression, epilepsy, fibrosis, inflammation, mastectomy patients, rheumatoid arthritis.

FUNCTIONS FACILITATED

Antioxidant, anti viral action, anti allergic properties, decreases inflammation, decreases vascular cell adhesion molecule expression, increases extravascular proteolysis through macrophages, induces eNOS, inhibits aldose reductase and keto reductase, inhibits angiogenesis, inhibits cancer proliferation by inducing apoptosis, inhibits lipoxygenase, cyclo-oxygenase, phospholipase A2 and xanthine oxidase; improves insulin function in diabetes, inhibits mast cell release of histamine, inhibits rouleaux formation, inhibits the enzyme methyl transferase and aldose reductase, metabolic enzyme modulator, prevents abnormal platelet adhesion, primes non specific immune system, protects vitamin C and adrenaline from oxidation, reduces blood sugar levels, reduces capillary fragility and permeability, reduces endothelial cell sloughing, stabilises lysosomal membranes, stimulates phase II detoxification reactions, strengthens capillaries.

SPECIFIC FUNCTIONS OF QUERCETIN

May be effective against ovarian, prostate and oestrogen receptor negative breast cancer, melanoma, and leukaemia.

Immune stimulator, anti-inflammatory action, free radical scavenger, alters mitotic cycle of tumour cells, modulates gene expression, anti-angiogenesis activity, induces apoptosis in tumour cells, modulates the activity of aldose reductase, phospholipase A2, cyclo-oxygenase (COX 1 & 2) and lipoxygenase; blocks GO/G1 phase in cellular division, binds to beta oestrogen receptors.

SPECIFIC FUNCTIONS OF RUTIN

Binds iron (metal chelator), inhibits 9-keto reductase, inhibits the effect of bradykinin on smooth muscle, improves abnormal erythrocyte deformability, prevents bruising, stabilises red blood cell membranes, inhibits rouleaux formation, reduces cytotoxicity of oxidised LDL-cholesterol, reduces venous oedema, reduces endothelial sloughing in the bloodstream, reduces erythema associated with X-rays, strengthens capillaries.

Flavonoids contribute to cancer prevention by:

- Free radical scavenging
- Detoxification of mutagens and xenobiotics
- Inhibition of topisomerase, cyclin dependant kinases
- Inhibits phosphatidyl-inositol-3-3kinase
- Inhibition of fatty acid synthase

DEFICIENCY MAY CAUSE OR BE ASSOCIATED WITH:

Bruising, capillary fragility diminished vitamin C activity, excessive inflammation, compromised immunity, purple and blue spots on skin.

THERAPEUTIC USES

Allergic conjunctivitis, allergy, atherosclerosis, arthritis, asthma, bleeding gums, bruising, burns, cancer, cataracts, cardiovascular disease, chronic pelvic pain syndrome in men, colds, diabetes, diabetic retinitis, emphysema, epilepsy, fibrosis, frost bite, glaucoma, haemorrhages, haemorrhoids, herpes (type 1), high blood pressure, high protein-oedema, infections, inflammation, lymphoedema, mastectomy patients, Meniere's disease, microvarices of the vocal cord, migraine, muscular degeneration, nose bleeds, pain (traumatic type), pancreatitis, post ischaemic oedema, prostatitis, radiotherapy, retinitis, schizophrenia, sinusitis, sprains, strokes, surgical trauma, varicose veins, viral infection (herpes, Epstein Barr's virus).

DAILY DOSAGE	
RDA	None stated
SR	600mg – 3g

EFFECTS OF OVERDOSAGE AND TOXICITY
None reported.

TECHNICAL NOTES

SYNERGISTIC NUTRIENTS

Vitamin B_6, C, E, coumarin (i.e. 5-6 benzopyrene), tyrosine, zinc.

OTHER POLYPHENOLS OF INTEREST

The flavonoids consist of 6 major subgroups: chalcone, flavone, flavonol, flavanone, anthocyanins and isoflavonoids.

Anthocyanins

Cyanidin, delphenidin, malvidin, pelargonidin.

Present in: bilberries, elderberries, gooseberries, mulberries, black currants, red grapes, raspberries, red cabbage, strawberries.

Anthocyanin supplementation may have a role in the prevention or treatment of chronic inflammatory diseases by inhibition of NF- B transactivation and deceased plasma concentrations of pro-inflammatory chemokines, cytokines, and inflammatory mediators.

Flavonols

Citrus bioflavonoids, quercetin, quercitrin (glycoside flavonol), myricetin, kaempferol.

Present in: onions, red grapes, cranberries, lemons, cocoa, buckwheat, blueberries and apple peel.

STRUCTURE OF QUERCETIN

STRUCTURE OF RUTIN

Rutin Structure: Rutoside, querce-tin-3-rutinoside Formula: $C_{27}H_{30}O_{16}$

Flavanols

Catechin, epicatechin, epigallocatechin-3-gallate, epicatechin gallate.

Present in: tea – black tea, oolong tea, green tea, cocoa.

Anti-tumour effect, inhibits angiogenesis and VEGF induced signalling, neuroprotective, antioxidant, prevents memory regression and DNA oxidation.

STRUCTURES OF GREEN TEA-DERIVED CATECHINS

R=H (-)-epicatechin (EC)
R=OH_1 (-)-epigallocatechin (EGC)

R=H (-)-epicatechin gallate (EC)
R=OH_1 (-)-epigallocatechin gallate (EGC)

Flavanones

Hesperetin, naringenin, reiodictyol, citrus bioflavinoids, hesperidin.

Present in citrus fruit.

Naringenin, an antioxidant flavanone from citrus species, has -OH groups attached at positions 5, 7, and 4'. Studies have indicated that it has anti-inflammatory, anti-cancer, and liver protective effects.

STRUCTURE OF NARINGENIN

Grape fruit juice contains nerigenin; which inhibits the breakdown of drug metabolising enzymes, thus increasing the risk of serious side effects.

Naringenin and drug interactions The following drugs are known to have potentially serious interactions:	
DRUG NAME	**TYPE OF DRUG**
Carbamazepine (Carbatrol, Tegretol)	An anti-seizure medication
Buspirone (BuSpar), clomipramine (Anafranil) and sertraline (Zoloft)	Antidepressants
Diazepam (Valium), triazolam (Halcion)	Tranquilizers
Felodipine (Plendil), nifedipine (Adalat, Procardia), nimodipine (Nimotop), nisoldipine (Sular) and possibly verapamil (Isoptin, Verelan)	Calcium channel blockers used to treat high blood pressure
Saquinavir (Invirase) and indinavir (Crixivan)	HIV medications
Simvastatin (Zocor), lovastatin (Mevacor, Altoprev) and atorvastatin (Lipitor), simvastatin-ezetimibe (Vytorin)	HMG-CoA reductase inhibitors used to treat high cholesterol
Cyclosporine (Neoral, Sandimmune), tacrolimus (Prograf) and sirolimus (Rapamune)	Immunosuppressant drugs
Amiodarone (Cordarone)	A drug used to treat and prevent abnormal heart rhythms (arrhythmias)
Methadone	Pain relief medication
Sildenafil (Viagra)	Erectile dysfunction medication

STRUCTURE OF HESPERIDIN

Flavones

Apigenin, luteolin, methoxy flavones – tangeretin, nibeiletin, sinensetin,

Present in: peel of citrus fruit, celery, parsley, sweet red peppers.

STRUCTURE OF FLAVONES

Name	R1	R2
Luteolin	OH	OH
Apigenin	H	OH
Diosmetin	OH	OCH3

Isoflavones

Daidzein, genistein, glycitin

Present: in soy products, red clover, alphaalpha, peas.

STRUCTURE OF GENISTEIN

Genistein

Genistein is protective against breast, prostate, and colon cancers and can help with hot flashes and osteoporosis prevention.

STRUCTURE OF DAIDZEIN

Daidzein

Anti-inflammatory properties, cardio-protective

THE MOLECULAR STRUCTURE OF EACH GROUP OF FLAVONOIDS

The flavones are characterized by a planar structure because of a double bond in the central aromatic ring. One of the best described flavonoids, quercetin, is a member of this group. Quercetin is found in abundance in onions, apples, broccoli, and berries.

The second group is the flavanones, which are mainly found in citrus fruit. An example of a flavonoid of this group is narigin.

Flavonoids belonging to the catechins are mainly found in green and black tea and in red wine, whereas anthocyanins are found in strawberries and other berries, grapes, wine, and tea.

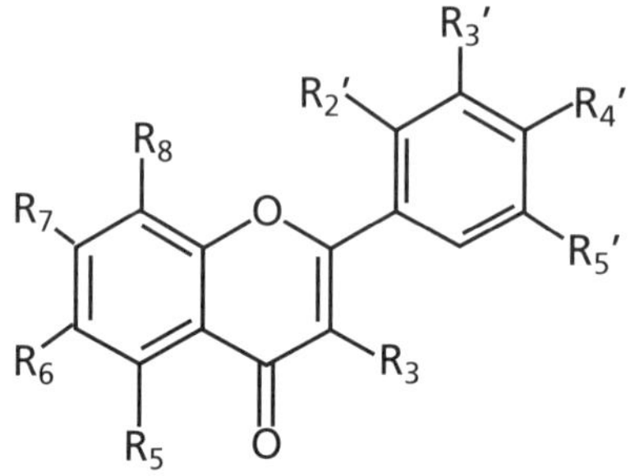

Flavone

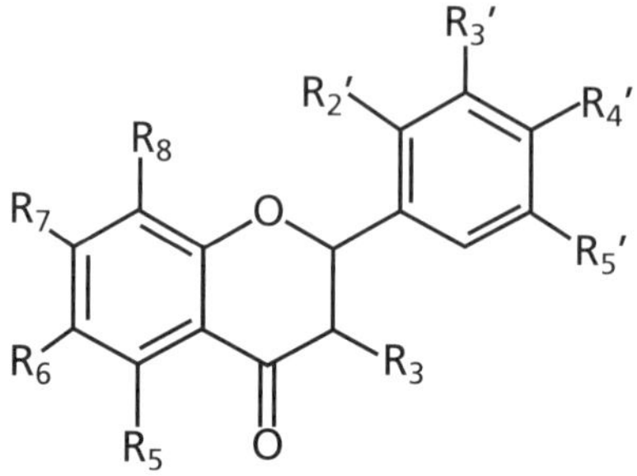

Flavanone

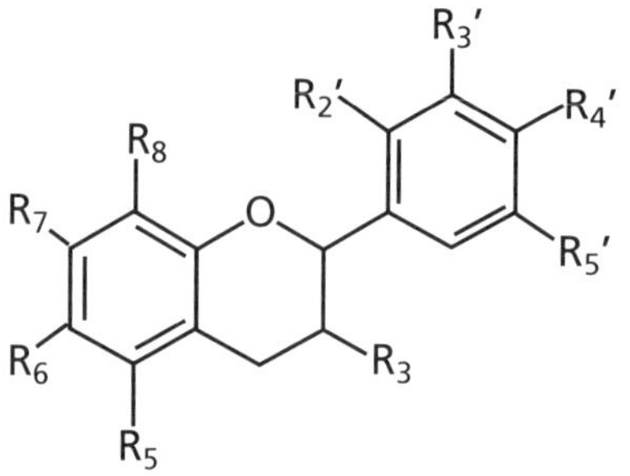

Catechin

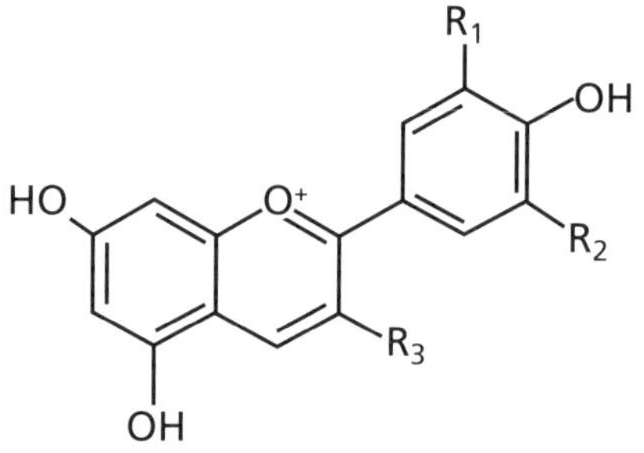

Anthocyanin

Biotin

(known as vitamin H or Co enzyme R)

SOURCE

Bacterial synthesis in gut, bean sprouts, butter, Bulgar wheat, cashews, egg yolk, kidney, liver, milk, oats, peanuts, soy beans, wholegrain cereals, yeast.

PROCESSING LOSSES

Unstable in acid and alkali solutions

Grain processing – 20-30%

Storage – 15%

FACTORS INCREASING DEMAND

Ageing, alcohol, anticonvulsant medication (carbamazepine, phenytoin), athletes, coffee, excess raw egg white intake, high lipoic acid intake, infant seborrhoeic dermatitis, lactation, pregnancy, propionic academia, surgical removal of stomach.

FUNCTIONS FACILITATED

Carboxylation reactions, decarboxylation reactions, deamination reactions, co-enzyme for carbon dioxide transfer, Co-factor for the following enzymes: acetyl CoA carboxylase (fatty acid synthesis), pyruvate carboxylase, methyl crotonyl CoA carboxylase and propionyl CoA carboxylase; cross linking of proteins in hair and nails, improves cardio metabolic risk factors, improves abnormal glucose metabolism, increases cellular cyclic GMP levels, induces epidermal differentiation, maintenance of skin, hair, sebaceous glands, bone marrow and sex glands; metabolism of fat, protein and sugars, cell growth, liver function; reduces cholesterol plaques on blood vessels, regulates glucokinase genetic expression, inhibits transcription of phosphoenolpyruvate carboxykinase.

DEFICIENCY MAY CAUSE OR BE ASSOCIATED WITH:

Alopecia, anaemia, anorexia, burning/tingling sensations, defects in T-cell and B-cell immunity, depression, dry greyish skin, extreme fatigue, glossitis, hallucinations, hyperaesthesia, hypercholesterolaemia, hypoglycaemia, increase in bile pigments and cholesterol, insomnia, ketosis, loss of hair colour, maculo-squamous dermatitis, mental depression, metabolic acidosis, muscle pain, nausea, pale smooth tongue, scaly and seborrhoeic dermatitis, scaly red rash distributed around the openings of eyes, mouth, nose and perianal areas; thinning of hair, increased excretion of 3-hydroxy isovaleric acid.

THERAPEUTIC USES

Diabetes (type I and II), diabetic peripheral neuropathy, acne, alcoholism, alopecia, anti-convulsant medication use, biotinidase deficiency, brittle nails, burning legs, burns and scalds, cholesterol plaques, dermatitis, diabetes, eczema, epileptics, holocarboxylase synthetase deficiency, hyperglycaemia, hyperlipidemia, lameness, leg cramps, propionic acidemia.

DAILY DOSES	
RDA	30-100 µg
Children 7-10 years of age	30 mcg per day
Children 4 to 6 years of age	25 mcg per day
Children birth-3 years of age	10 to 20 mcg per day
SR	0.5-15 mg

RDA by age:	
0 – 0.5 yrs	10 µg
0.5 – 1 yrs	15 µg
1 – 3 yrs	20 µg
7 – 10 yrs	30 µg
4 – 6 yrs	25 µg
>11 yrs	30-300 µg

EFFECTS OF OVERDOSAGE AND TOXICITY

Essentially non-toxic to humans.

TECHNICAL NOTES

SYNERGISTIC NUTRIENTS

Bifidobacterium, chromium. Vitamin B_2, B_3, B_5, B_6, B_{12}, folate, magnesium, manganese.

TARGET TISSUES

Bone marrow, kidney, liver, male genitalia, nervous tissue, skin.

DRUG/NUTRIENT INTERACTIONS

Decrease gut synthesis of biotin:
Antibiotics – Aminoglycosides, Cephalosporins, Fluoroquinolones, Quinolones, Macrolides, Penicillins, Sulfonamides, Tetracyclines, Trimethoprin-containing antibiotics, Carbapenems, Monobactams, chloramphenicol, spectinomycin, Streptogramins, vancomycin, Oxalodinones, Lincosamides, Nitrofurans.

Lower body biotin levels:
Anticonvulsant drugs – phenytoin, carbamazepine, primidone, gabapentin, valproic acid, felbamate, lamotrigine, mephenytoin, fosphenytoin, clonazepam, ethosuximide, diazepam, clorazepate dipotassium, levatiracetam, tiagabine, topiramate, methsuximide, phensuximide, trimethadione, magnesium sulfate, acetazolamide, oxcarbazepine, zonisamide, ethotoin.

Alcohol, Cephalosporin, Doxycycline.

ENZYME SYSTEMS INVOLVED

Carboxylases e.g. pyruvate carboxylase, acetyl-Co A carboxylase.

DEFICIENCY SYMPTOMS AS RELATED TO METABOLIC ACTION	
Skin disorders	Decreased fatty acid synthesis, decreased synergism with vitamins A, D, and B complex.
Hyperaesthesia	Increased lactic acid levels.
Fatigue and somnolence	Decreased oxidation of pyruvate.
Muscle pain	Increased lactic acid levels, decreased fatty acid synthesis, burning legs

STRUCTURE OF BIOTIN

Biotin

Biotin is a prosthetic group of enzymes involved in carboxylation (e.g., pyruvate carboxylase).

Vitamin C

Ascorbic Acid

SOURCE

Aloe vera juice, blackcurrant, broccoli, brussel sprouts, citrus fruit, guava, parsley, pawpaw, peppers, pineapple, potatoes, raw cabbage, rosehips, strawberries, sweet potatoes, tomatoes.

PROCESSING LOSSES

Unstable to heat, light and alkali
Losses during processing 10-90%

FACTORS INCREASING DEMAND

Achlorhydria, acute or chronic inflammatory conditions, AIDS, allergies, antimicrobial therapy, arthritis, atherosclerosis, athletic performance, burns, cancer, cold and heat stress, diabetes, drug toxicity, exercise, exposure to DDT and dieldrin, heavy metal intoxication, hemodialysis, hyperglycaemia, hypertension, infection (prolonged), intestinal disease, lactation, periodontal disease, pregnancy, pressure sores, nitrate exposure, radium therapy, scar tissue, smokers, stress, surgery, thyrotoxicosis, tuberculosis.

FUNCTIONS FACILITATED

Antihistamine properties, antioxidant, blood cell formation, bone and teeth growth, collagen synthesis, decreases mRNA levels of apolipoprotein A1, detoxifies toxic metabolites, essential for healthy teeth and gums, excretion of heavy metals, fibrolytic agents, hydroxylation reactions, hydroxylation of prolyl and lysyl, residues of procollagen, improves immunity, improves sperm motility, inhibits phosphodiesterase, maintains the integrity of connective tissue, osteoid tissue and dentin, maintenance of cell membranes, adrenals and ovaries, promotes healing, protects folic acid reductase, protects against nitrite and benzo-pyrene ingestion, reduces tumour metastasis, regulates cholesterol metabolism, wound healing, stimulates alpha hydroxylation of cholesterol by liver cytochrome P450.

DEFICIENCY MAY CAUSE OR BE ASSOCIATED WITH:

Abnormal brain function, abnormal drug metabolism, abnormal osteoid and dentin formation, bleeding gums, bulbar conjunctivitis, bruising easily, coiled hair, increased wound healing time, depression, fatigue, greater susceptibility to infection, haematomas, haemorrhage, hypercholesterolaemia, hypochondria, hysteria, increased risk of bladder, cervical, colorectal, oesophageal, lung and prostate cancer; lassitude, listlessness, malaise, myalgia and arthralgia, pains in joints, reduced work capacity, rough skin, scurvy, thrombosis, weakness, weight loss.

Scurvy symptoms in adults include: loss of appetite, diarrhea, shortness of breath, weakness, and fever, followed by irritability, depression, leg pain, pseudoparalysis, swelling over long bones of the body, anemia, paleness, poor wound healing, corkscrew hair, dry eyes, skin thickening (hyperkeratosis), and bleeding (particularly gum bleeding, bleeding behind the eyes causing prominence (proptosis), bleeding at the joints of the ribs and sternum causing discoloration under the skin of the chest (costochondral beading, scorbutic rosary), skin bruising, or blood in the urine or stool).

In infants: irritability, thigh tenderness, pseudoparalysis, bleeding around the lower ends of the leg bones (femur and tibia) causing pain, and assumption of a frog-leg posture. If left untreated, scurvy can proceed to seizures, shock or sudden death.

THERAPEUTIC USES

Alcoholism, allergies, anaemia, asthma exercised induced, atherosclerosis, athletes, bone fractures, burns, bursitis, cancer, cataracts, cervical dysplasia, colds, constipation, coronary thrombosis, Crohn's disease, degenerative vascular disease, depression, diabetes, drug toxicity, dry mouth, exposure to pollutants, headaches, heart disease, high blood cholesterol, high blood histamine, hyperglycaemia, hypertension, infection, infertility, inflammation, lactation, macular degeneration, moodiness, nitrate exposure, osteoarthritis, Parkinson's disease, periodontal disease, pregnancy, premature infants, pressure sores, prickly heat, reduces risk of a number of cancers including bladder, cervical, colorectal, oesophageal, lung, prostate, stomach and salivary gland cancer, leukaemia and non-Hodgkin's lymphoma; smokers, strenuous exercise, stress, sun burn, surgery, tobacco smoke exposure, tooth decay, trauma, vascular fragility, wound healing.

DAILY DOSAGE	
RDA	75-125 mg
SR	250-2000 mg Doses higher than 2 gm can be used to treat cancer (10-40gm have been used depending on the cancer)
Infants	40 mg
Children (1-3yrs)	50 mg

Tolerable Upper Intake Levels (UL) for vitamin C: Children ages:	
1-3 years-old	400 mg/day
4-8 years-old	650 mg/day
9-13 years-old	1200 mg/day
14-18 years-old	1800 mg/day (including pregnant or breastfeeding females).

Lipoic acid can reduce vitamin C requirements.

Deficiency signs occur when ascorbic acid levels in white blood cell-platelet layers drop below 2 µg/108 cells or <11.4 nmol/108 cells.

Fasting blood ascorbic acid levels below 0.10 mg/dL are considered deficient; levels of 0.10-0.19 mg/dL are considered low; levels of 0.2 mg/dL or greater are generally considered acceptable; and levels greater than 0.6 mg/dL likely rule out scurvy.

White blood cell ascorbic acid concentration is considered a more accurate measurement of vitamin C nutritional status, with a level of zero suggesting scurvy; 0-7 mg/dL suggesting deficiency; 8-15 mg/dL considered low; and 15 mg/dL or greater consistent with adequate vitamin C status.

Allergies, diarrhoea, gastritis, nausea, stomach cramps.

Enhances the absorption of aluminium – should not be taken with aluminium containing substances, possible kidney stones in individuals with gout.

Parenteral (injected) vitamin C may cause dizziness, faintness, injection site discomfort.

High doses of vitamin C should be avoided in people with conditions aggravated by acid loading, such as: cirrhosis, gout, renal tubular acidosis, or paroxysmal nocturnal hemoglobinuria.

High doses of vitamin C may cause hemolytic anemia in Glucose-6-phosphate dehydrogenase (G6PD) deficiency.

TECHNICAL NOTES

SYNERGISTIC NUTRIENTS

Vitamin A, B_5, B_6, B_{12}, E, calcium, copper, folate, iron, lipoic acid, lysine, magnesium, manganese, methionine, phosphorus, selenium, zinc.

Bioflavonoids increase the absorption of vitamin C by 35%.

DRUG/NUTRIENT INTERACTIONS

Aspirin, barbiturates, cimetidine, copper excess, cyclophosphamide, deoxy-corticosteroids, fluorouracil, oestrogen.

Acetaminophen – vitamin C decreases its excretion

Aspirin – vitamin C increases its excretion

Loop diuretics (furosemide) – vitamin C amplifies its effects

Beta blockers – decreases their absorption

Cyclosporin – decreases vitamin C levels in the blood

Nitrate drugs (nitroglycerin, isosorbide, dinitrate) – Vitamin C reduces the development of tolerance to these drugs

Tetracycline – vitamin C increases blood levels of this drug

Increase Vitamin C excretion:
   Salicylates – aspirin, choline salicylate, sodium salicylate, magnesium salicylate, salsalate, diflunisal, sodium thiosalicylate
   Loop diuretics – furosemide, bumetanide, ethacrynic acid, torsemide

Decrease cellular uptake of vitamin C in certain tissues:
   Corticosteroid medications – prednisone, hydrocortisone, methylprednisolone, prednisolone, betamethasone, budesonide, triamcinolone, dexamethasone, cortisone, beclomethasone, flunisolide, fluticasone, fludrocortisone, mometasone

Decrease vitamin C status:
   Oral contraceptives – norethindrone, ethynodiol diacetate, norgestrel, norgestimate, ethinyl estradiol, drospirenone, desogestrel, levonorgestrel

Decrease blood levels of vitamin C:
   Tetracyclines – tetracycline, demeclocycline, doxycycline, minocycline, oxytetracycline

NUTRIENT/NUTRIENT INTERACTIONS

High doses of **vitamin C** may decrease the absorption of copper from the digestive tract.

TARGET TISSUE

Adrenal cortex, bone, connective tissue, gums, liver, leucocytes, ovary, pituitary, teeth.

ENZYME SYSTEMS INVOLVED

Activates enzymes involved in proline, tryptophan, carnitine and steroid synthesis.

Activates many liver enzymes – amidases, catalase, cathepsin, cytochrome, esterases, peroxidase, and proteases.

DEFICIENCY SYMPTOMS AS RELATED TO METABOLIC ACTION	
Scurvy haemorrhages	Decreased synthesis of mucopolysaccharides, collagen synthesis.
Lethargy	Decreased supply of adreno-cortical and adrenal hormone.
Oedema	Decreased aldosterone synthesis and capillary fragility.
Infection	Decreased phagocytic activity and motility of white blood cells.

STRUCTURE VITAMIN C/ASCORBIC ACID

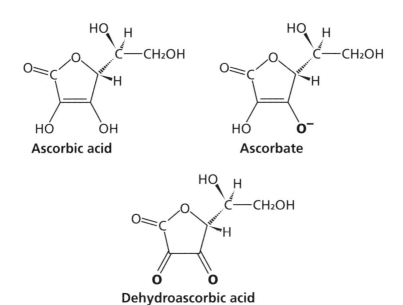

Ascorbic acid

Ascorbate

Dehydroascorbic acid

Choline

SOURCE

Beans, beef liver, chicken liver, egg yolk, lecithin, lentils, liver, milk, peanuts, split peas, soybeans, spinach, wholegrain cereals, yeast.

FACTORS INCREASING DEMAND

Alcohol & coffee consumption, liver disease, low protein diets, memory deficits.

FUNCTIONS FACILITATED

Detoxification of chemicals, formation of acetylcholine, co-ordination, muscle contraction, involved in betaine metabolism, methylation reactions, protection against the toxic effects of dl-methionine, regulation of fats and cholesterol, reduces blood cholesterol, plays an important role in cell membrane structure, myelin sheath integrity, memory enhancement and attention, synthesis of lecithin and sphingomyelin, lipotropic source of labile methyl groups, transport and metabolism of fats.

Increases the sensitivity of CA1 hippocampal neurons to long-term potentiation i.e. improves the laying down of long-term memory.

DEFICIENCY MAY CAUSE OR BE ASSOCIATED WITH:

Abnormal platelet aggregation, cirrhosis, elevated free radical damage in heart, kidney & liver; fatty liver, gastric ulcer, haemorrhage of kidney, adrenals and heart; hardening of arteries, hepatic carcinogenesis, increased blood pressure, impaired immune response, liver tumours, memory loss, panic/anxiety, poor neural tube closure, poor hippocampal development, reduced gene methylation, vascular damage.

THERAPEUTIC USES

Alcoholism, Alzheimer's disease, ataxia, atherosclerosis, cancer, carcinogen exposure, chorea, drug toxicity, gallbladder problems, glaucoma, headaches, high blood cholesterol, hypertension, Huntington's disease, infant growth, liver and colon cancer, mania, memory deficits, myasthenia gravis, pregnancy, schizophrenia, sympathetic dominance, tardive dyskinesia.

DAILY DOSAGE		
RDA	Adult male	550 mg
	Adult female	425 mg
	Pregnancy	600 mg
	Lactation	550 mg
SR	1-3.5 gm	

EFFECTS OF OVERDOSAGE AND TOXICITY

Depression, diarrhoea, dizziness, nausea, salivation.

SYNERGISTIC NUTRIENTS

Vitamins B_5, B_6, B_{12}, betaine, dimethyl glycine, ethanolamine, folic acid, inositol, methionine.

DRUG INTERACTIONS
Methotrexate

STRUCTURE OF CHOLINE

$$CH_3$$
$$|$$
$$CH_3 - N^+ - CH_2 - CH_3 - OH$$
$$|$$
$$CH_3$$

Choline

Vitamin D

1, 25-Dihydroxycholecalciferol (1,25-(OH)2 D3) (calcitriol or vitamin D hormone active form of the vitamin), Vitamin D2 (ergocalciferol) Vitamin D3 (cholecalciferol)- Prohormone

SOURCE

Synthesized by the action of sunlight on skin.

Fish liver oils – cod, halibut, herring, tuna, butter, egg yolk, milk, sprouted seeds.

PROCESSING LOSSES

Unstable to light

FACTORS INCREASING DEMAND

Alcohol, autoimmune reactive arthritis, bile problems, cancer (breast, prostate, colon and skin), Crohn's disease, cystic fibrosis, darked- skinned people, elderly individuals, hypoparathyroidism, intestinal disorders, insulin dependent diabetes, kidney disorders, lack of exposure to sun, lactation, liver disease, mineral oil intake, multiple sclerosis, obesity, pancreatic disease, pregnancy, rickets, schizophrenia, smog exposure, ulcerative colitis, use of anti convulsants e.g. phenytoin and phenobarbitol, steroid medication, vegetarianism.

SITE OF ACTION

Activated lymphocytes, bone, haematopoietic cells, intestine, keratinocytes of the skin, kidney, pancreatic islet cells, parathyroid hormone, reproductive organs, and thymus T cells.

INDICATIONS

Diabetes, heart failure (congestive), heart transplants, leukaemia, multiple sclerosis, psoriasis, rheumatoid arthritis.

FUNCTIONS FACILITATED

Antiproliferative effect – osteosarcoma, melanoma, colon and breast cancer, apoptosis, blood clotting, calcium and phosphate absorption and regulation, cofactor in synthesis of heat shock proteins, differentiates leukemic cells and induces apoptosis, heart and muscle action, helps induce monocyte conversion to macrophages, increases bone strength, induces apoptosis in breast and prostate cancer, increases neurotrophic factor synthesis (NGF, GDNF, NF-3), increases the activity of tyrosine hydroxylase and choline acetyl transferase, increases neural glutathione levels, inhibits iNOS and TNF – alpha activity, mineralisation of bone and teeth, potent antiproliferative agent in the colon, protects against neurotoxicity associated with ischaemia, regulates cellular differentiation in intestinal cells, regulates or inhibits T-cell mediated immune responses, regulation of calcium and phosphorus metabolism, selectively reduces interleukin 2 levels and proliferation of T cells, stimulates polyamine and heat shock protein synthesis, stimulator of ornithine decarboxylase and spermidine acetyl transferase.

DEFICIENCY MAY CAUSE OR BE ASSOCIATED WITH:

Burning in the mouth and throat, cramps, diabetes (type 1), diarrhoea, hyperparathyroidism, increased serum phosphatase, increases in FSH and LH production, insomnia, low birth weight, myopia, nervousness, osteomalacia, osteoporosis, retarded growth, rickets, skeletal abnormalities, softening of bones and teeth.

THERAPEUTIC USES

Acute leukaemia, arthritis, astrocytoma, autism, autoimmune encephalomyelitis, autoimmune disease, bone fractures, breast cancer, carpopedal spasm, cerebral palsy, chronic renal failure, coeliac disease, colorectal cancer, convulsion, Crohn's disease, diabetes (type 1), diabetes (type II), gliomas, graft rejection, hyperparathyroidism, hypertension, inflammatory bowel disease, juvenile arthritis, lactation, laryngospasm, Lyme disease, muscle weakness, multiple sclerosis, neuromuscular irritability, oestrogen sensitive breast metastasis, osteomalacia, obesity, osteoporosis, pregnancy, prostate cancer, psoriasis (topically applied), rheumatoid arthritis, rickets, low exposure to sun, Syndrome X, tetany, ulcerative colitis.

DAILY DOSAGE

(Note: 40 IU = 1 µg vitamin D [active form])

RDA	200-400 IU
SR	400-3000 IU

Or 2000-8000 IU/day (50-200 µg/day) for three weeks.

RDA by age:	
0 – 0.5 yrs	7.5 µg (300 IU)
1 – 24 yrs	10 µg (400 IU)
>24 yrs	5 µg (200 IU)
>60 yrs	25 µg (1000 IU)

The daily "upper limit" for vitamin D is 25 micrograms (1,000 IU) for infants up to 12 months of age and 50 micrograms (2,000 IU) for children, adults, pregnant, and lactating women, due to toxicities that can occur when taken in higher doses.

Taking vitamin D with fructose will lower phosphate levels and increase circulating vitamin D levels. Lycopene and vitamin D work synergistically in reducing tumour proliferation.

Do not give to sarcoidosis patients.
Sarcoidosis patients synthesise vitamin D or calcitriol within inflammatory granuloma by macrophages, under the influence of angiotensin II and interferon gamma. While most sarcoidosis patients posses high blood levels of vitamin D, they do not exhibit hypercalcaemia.

Levels of > 42 pg/ml stimulate bone osteoclasts, causing bone resorption and osteoporosis, calcium precipitation in the soft tissues of the lung, breasts and kidneys.

EFFECTS OF OVERDOSAGE AND TOXICITY

Vitamin D 1000 µg (40,000 IU)/day produces toxicity within 1-4 months in infants and as little as 75 µg (3,000 IU)/day can produce toxicity over years. Serum calcium levels are elevated 12-16 mg/dl as compared to 8.5-10.5 mg/dl in normal adults. Blood levels > 45 pg/ml indicates toxicity.

Early symptoms of hypercalcemia may include: nausea, vomiting, and anorexia (appetite/weight loss), followed by polyuria (excess urination), polydipsia (excess thirst), weakness, fatigue, somnolence, headache, anorexia, dry mouth, metallic taste, vertigo, tinnitus (ear ringing), and ataxia (unsteadiness). Kidney function may become impaired, and metastatic calcifications (calcium deposition in organs throughout the body) may occur, particularly affecting the kidneys.

$1,25(OH)_2D_3$ is 100 times more potent than vitamin D3 (cholcalciferol).

Treat vitamin D toxicity with low calcium diets and keep the urine acidic.

Dosages of more than 100,00 IU or 2500 μg – anorexia, arteriosclerosis, asthenia, cardiomyopathy and/or renal failure, diarrhoea, headache, hypercalcaemia, joint pain, kidney damage, metastatic calcification in kidneys, muscle weakness or pain, nausea, polydipsia, proteinuria, precipitation of calcium in tissues, polyuria, skin rash, thirst.

In sarcoidosis patients, as little as 9000 IU can trigger exacerbation of sarcoidosis.

TECHNICAL NOTES

SYNERGISTIC NUTRIENTS

Vitamin A, B_3, K, boron, calcium, copper lycopene, manganese, magnesium, phosphorus, silica, sodium.

Excess calcium intake may decrease production of vitamin D, and result in increased risk of autoimmunity, sarcoidosis, diabetes and cancers.

Vitamin A optimizes Vitamin D action.

DRUG/NUTRIENT INTERACTIONS

Interfere with vitamin D metabolism:
Anticonvulsants – phenytoin, carbamazepine, primidone, gabapentin, valproic acid, felbamate, lamotrigine, mephenytoin, fosphenytoin, clonazepam, ethosuximide, diazepam, clorazepate dipotassium, levatiracetam, tiagabine, topiramate, methsuximide, phensuximide, trimethadione, magnesium sulfate, acetazolamide, oxcarbazepine, zonisamide, ethotoin

Corticosteroid medications – prednisone, hydrocortisone, methylprednisolone, prednisolone, betamethasone, budesonide, triamcinolone, dexamethasone, cortisone, beclomethasone, flunisolide, fluticasone, fludrocortisone, mometasone
Cimetidine

Decrease absorption of Vitamin D:
Bile acid sequestrants – cholestyramine, colestipol, colesevelam
Mineral oil

Decrease body vitamin D status:
Isoniazid, Rifampin, Orlistat, Cyclosporine, Leflunomide, Mycophenolate, Mofetil, Neomycin, Phenobarbitol.

Vitamin D acts synergistically with hormone suppression drugs.

TARGET TISSUES

Bone, intestine, kidney, liver. In the liver, vitamin D_3 is converted to $25(OH)D_3$ and the kidney then further hydroxylates it to $1,25(OH)_2D_3$.

Vitamin D receptors are present in all tissues and cells.

ENZYME SYSTEMS INVOLVED

- Acts like a steroid hormone through receptor-mediated regulation of nuclear events.
- Increases intracellular cGMP.
- Activates alkaline phosphatase, phosphorylase.

DEFICIENCY SYMPTOMS AS RELATED TO METABOLIC ACTION

Decreased growth and skeletal abnormalities	retarded calcification and bone growth.
Differentiation of cells	stimulates polyamine synthesis.
Increased alkaline phosphatase	attempt by the body to increase phosphate.
Osteomalacia	demineralisation of bone, deficient synthesis of bone GLA protein and matrix GLA protein.

STRUCTURE OF VITAMIN D AND VARIOUS ANALOGUES

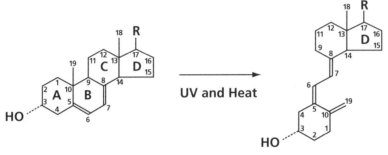

Vitamin D [1α25 (OH)₂ D3]
Calcitriol

UV and Heat

Provitamin D
7-Dehydrocholesterol

Vitamin D3
Cholecalciferol

R= **D₂**

R= **D**

R= **D**

R= **D**

R= **D**

R= **D**

Various Analogues

Vitamin E

Tocopherol (There are 8 naturally occurring compounds that can be divided into two classes – tocopherols and tocotrienols)

SOURCE

Almonds, apricot oil, beef, corn, egg yolk, hazel nuts, safflowers, sunflowers, wheat germ.

PROCESSING LOSSES

Sensitive to alkali, heat, light

Milling of flour – 80%

FACTORS INCREASING DEMAND

Apo E_4 gene types, athletes, beta thalassemia, cancer, cardiomyopathy, chronic cholestatic hepatobiliary disease, coeliac disease, Crohn's disease, cystic fibrosis, Crohn's diease, diabetes, ageing, epileptic drugs, excess intake of polyunsaturated oil, exposure to air pollutants, extrahepatic biliary atresia, heart disease, hyper-oestrogenism, lactation, lead toxicity, liver and gall bladder disease, methyl mercury poisoning, malabsorption syndromes, mitochondrial lesions, pancreatic dysfunction, pregnancy, premature infants, radiation or radium therapy, short bowel syndrome, smoking, vascular fragility.

FUNCTIONS FACILITATED

Intracellular antioxidant, reduces synthesis or release of interleukin 1B, lipid soluble antioxidant, enhances T helper cell synthesis, inhibits protein kinase-C and 5-lipoxygenase, activates protein phosphatase 2A and diacyl-glycerol kinase, inhibits platelet aggregation and monocyte adhesion, inhibits cell proliferation, immune modulator, traps peroxyl radicals, maintains lipid membrane integrity, modulates liver collagen alpha gene & collagenase gene, modulates the activity of cyclo-oxygenase, lipoxygenase & phospholipase; prevents tissue polyunsaturated fatty acid peroxidation, regulates synthesis of sex hormones, represses the synthesis of xanthine oxidase and creatine kinase, required for superoxide dismutase function, stabilises cell membranes, improves blood flow, stabilises normal growth maintenance, fertility and gestation, reduces cognitive decline in the elderly.

Reduces the toxicity (calcium overload) of vitamin D.

All forms of vitamin E activate a gene expansion via Pregnane X receptor (PXP); a nuclear receptor which regulates a variety of drug metabolising genes.

Tocopheryl succinate:
Dosage: 400-800 mg/day

- Induces apoptosis in many cancer cell lines. e.g. prostate, breast, lung, colon, gastric cancer.
- Increases Fas and Fas L expression.
- Inhibits endothelial growth factor gene expression.
- Inhibits angiogenesis.
- Improves Transforming Growth Factor b (TGF-b) signalling.
- Regulates protein kinase-C in smooth muscle walls.
- Mitochondrial targeted anti-cancer drug.

Gamma tocopherol:
- Quenches peroxynitrite free radicals.
- Inhibits an enzyme that promotes cholesterol plaque formation.
- Reduces inflammation.

DEFICIENCY MAY CAUSE OR BE ASSOCIATED WITH:

Areflexia, ceroid deposition in muscle, cardiomyopathy, chronic liver disease, cirrhosis of the gall bladder, creatinuria, cystic fibrotic symptoms, diminished proprioception, gait disturbances, involuntary eye movements, kyphoscoliosis, muscle wasting and weakness, nerve damage, neuromuscular deficits, platelet hyperaggregability, poor immunity, poor coordination, pulmonary embolism, red blood cell haemolysis, red blood cell fragility, reno lytic anaemia, shortened RBC half-life, spinocerebellar disease.

Familiar Vitamin E Deficiency Symptoms
Ataxia, altered proprioception and vibratory sense, absent deep tendon reflex, Babinski's sign, cardiomyopathy, kyphoscoliosis, dysarthria.

THERAPEUTIC USES
Ageing, air pollution, Alzheimer's disease, angina, arthritis, atherosclerosis, auto immune disease, Bayler's disease (intrahepatic cholestasis), blood clots, burns, broncho pulmonary dysplasia, cancer therapy (tocopheryl succinate form), cataracts, cardiomyopathy, chemical sensitive individuals, cholestatic liver disease, coeliac disease, congenital atresia (gall bladder), cystic fibrosis, cystic mastitis, diabetes, epilepsy, exercise induced peroxidation, external scars, fibrocystic breast disease, heart disease, infection, infertility, inflammation, intermittent claudication, involuntary eye movements, macular degeneration, menstrual problems, multiple sclerosis, muscle cramps, muscular dystrophy, neuromuscular dysfunction associated with malabsorption, ozone exposure, Parkinson's disease, platelet aggregation, premenstrual tension, respiratory distress syndrome, retrolental fibroplasia, rheumatoid arthritis, sickle cell anaemia, sinusitis, steatohepatitis, stroke, tardive dyskinesia, thalassemia major, thrombosis, varicose veins, very low birth weight babies, wound healing.

Tocopherol succinate:
Angiogenesis, breast cancer, prostate cancer, tumour growth.

Gamma tocopherol
Asthma, rheumatoid arthritis, high nitric oxide conditions, inflammation.

DAILY DOSAGE of Tocopherol (Vitamin E)	
RDA	30 mg
SR	100 – 800 mg
Infant	10 mg
Children (1-3yrs)	15 mg

Plasma levels associated with deficiency – <5 µg/ml or <11.6 µmol/l. However, if hyperlipidemia is present, <7 µg/ml is considered deficient.

EFFECTS OF OVERDOSAGE AND TOXICITY
Allergy, fatigue, general dermatitis (in a few individuals). May increase blood cholesterol and lipids.
>3000 mg/day increases fragility of red blood cells, decreased antimicrobial activity of white blood cells.

TECHNICAL NOTES

SYNERGISTIC NUTRIENTS
Vitamin A, B_2, B_6, B_{12}, C, K, copper, cysteine, folic acid, glutathione, iron, lipoic acid, manganese, phosphorus, potassium, selenium, sodium and zinc. Gamma tocopherol improves the activity of d-alpha tocopherol; mixed tocopherols.

Decreases blood levels of vitamin E:
Gemfibrozil

Decreases liver vitamin E levels:
Fenofibrate

Decrease body vitamin E status:
Haloperidol Adriamycin, Alpha
Tocopherol Quinone, Aspirin, Epileptic
Drugs, Iron, Nitrofurantoin, Oral
Contraceptives, Oxidants, Thyroxine

Anticoagulant medications: warfarin,
heparin, dalteparin, tinzaparin, enoxaparin, danaparoid sodium, antithrombin
III, lipirudin, argatroban, bivalirudin.

Potential/Theoretical Risk: Vitamin E
may increase the bleeding effect of these
medications when taken in high doses.
Vitamin E can also increase blood clotting
time. Therefore, taking high doses of this
vitamin is not advised for individuals
taking anticoagulant drugs.

NUTRIENT/NUTRIENT INTERACTIONS

**Polyunsaturated fatty acids (PUFAs)
– Omega-3 and omega-6 fatty acids,
cod liver oil.** High intakes of PUFAs can
decrease vitamin E levels in the body or
increase requirement for the vitamin.

Chitosan – the absorption of fat-soluble
nutrients, such as vitamin E, from the
digestive tract. It is recommended not to
take these agents at the same time.

TARGET TISSUES

Adrenals, bone marrow, brain, genital
organs, kidneys, liver, lungs, muscles,
pituitary.

ENZYME SYSTEMS INVOLVED

Indirect action by way of the maintenance
of reducing conditions or redox poten-
tials and stabilisation of cell membranes.
Improves activity of glutathione and selenium, and superoxide dismutase.

DEFICIENCY SYMPTOMS AS RELATED TO METABOLIC ACTION	
Creatinuria and muscular dystrophy	maintenance of muscle cell membranes.
Poor immunity and inflammation	prostaglandin synthesis and regulation.
Red blood cell haemolysis	maintenance of red cell membranes.

Tocotrienols

SOURCE

Palm oil, rice oil, barley oil, almonds, pistachio nuts.

FUNCTIONS FACILITATED

Acts as antioxidant, Inhibits tumour angiogenesis, decreases cholesterol, inhibits lipid peroxidation, inhibits nuclear factor kappa B activation, inhibits monocyte adhesion to endothelium, counteracts the free radicals produced by excessive sun exposure, inhibits activity of protein kinase-C (PKC), inhibits production and activity of HMG-CoA reductase, lowers elevated cholesterol levels, neuroprotective, prevents side effects of long term glucocorticoid use (increases calcium content of bones), protects against glutamate induced neuronal death, suppresses inducible 12-lipoxygenase activation, reduces VCAM 1 expression. Tocotrienols up-regulate endogenous CYP3A4, CYP3A5 mRNA.

THERAPEUTIC USES

Atherosclerosis, Alzheimer's disease; angiogenic disorders – tumour growth, diabetic retinopathy, rheumatoid arthritis; Breast cancer, liver cancer, skin cancer, melanoma, high cholesterol, long term glucocorticoid use, stroke associated brain damage.

DAILY DOSAGE	
SR 100	160mg/day

STRUCTURE OF VITAMIN E AND TOCOTRIENOLS

Vitamin E
Tocopherol

A

α-Tocopherol

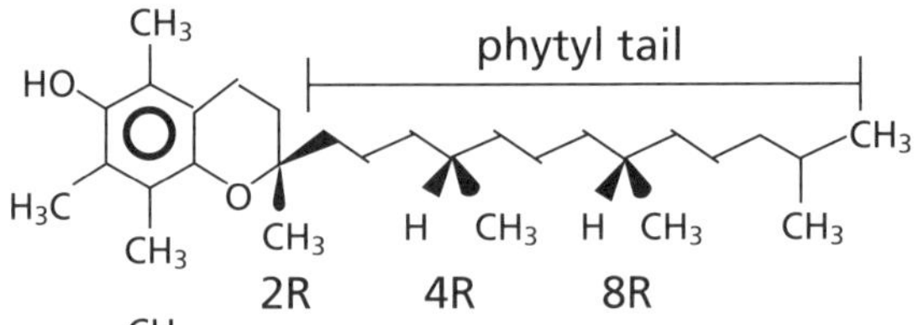

phytyl tail

CH₃

HO

H₃C

CH₃ CH₃ H CH₃ H CH₃ CH₃

2R 4R 8R

β-Tocopherol

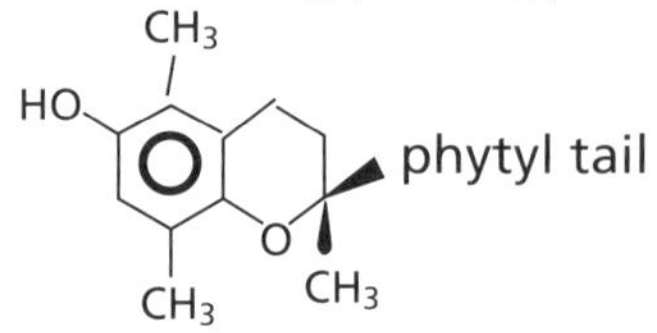

CH₃

HO

phytyl tail

CH₃ CH₃

γ-Tocopherol

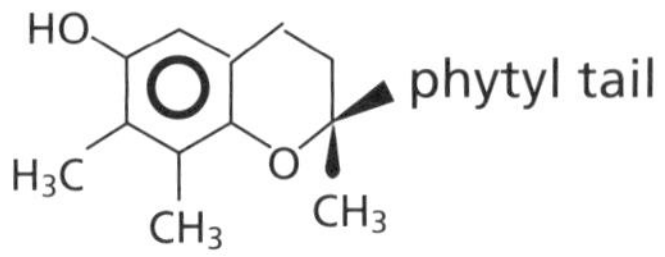

HO

phytyl tail

H₃C

CH₃ CH₃

δ-Tocopherol

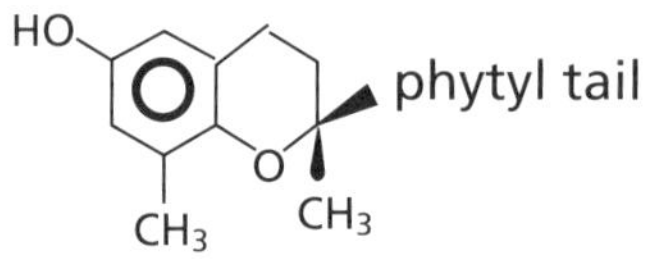

HO

phytyl tail

CH₃ CH₃

B

α-Tocotrienol

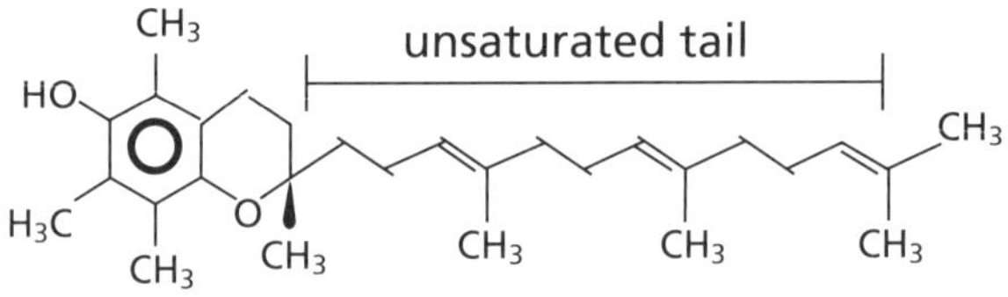

CH₃

HO

unsaturated tail

CH₃

H₃C

CH₃ CH₃ CH₃ CH₃ CH₃

β-Tocotrienol

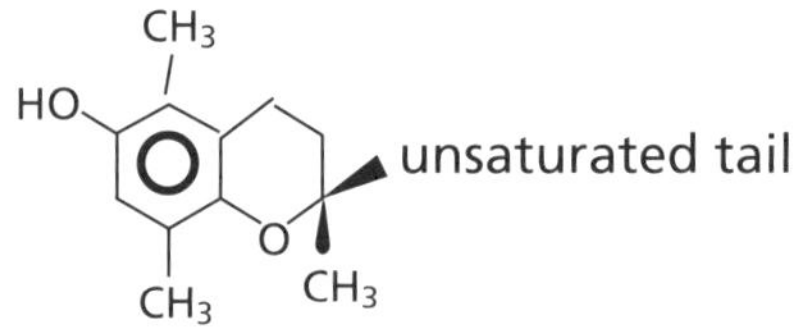

CH₃

HO

unsaturated tail

CH₃ CH₃

γ-Tocotrienol

HO

unsaturated tail

H₃C

CH₃ CH₃

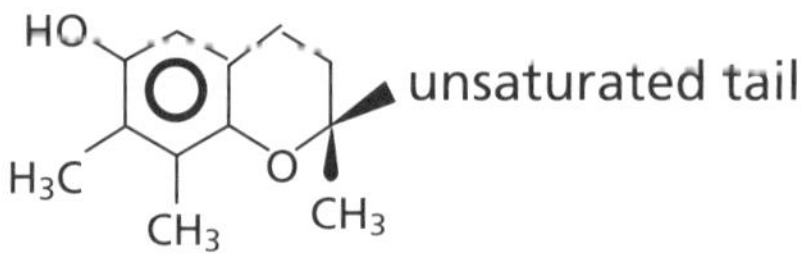

δ-Tocotrienol

HO

unsaturated tail

CH₃ CH₃

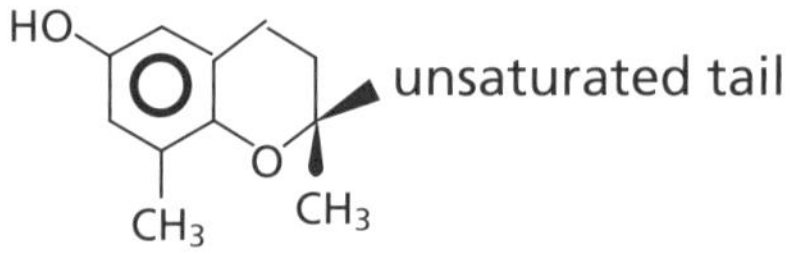

Essential Fatty Acids

ACTIVE COMPONENTS

Linoleic acid, linolenic acid, conjugated linoleic acid (cis9/trans11 and trans10/cis12 isomers [CLA]), gamma linolenic acid (GLA), arachidonic acid (AA), eicosapentaenoic acid (EPA), docosahexaenoic acid (DHA).

SOURCE

Butternuts, corn oil, evening primrose oil, purslane, rapeseed oil, seaweed, sunflower oil, tofu, walnut oil, wheat germ oil.

Omega-3 – cod liver oil, mustard seed oil, linseed oil, tuna, salmon and cod, walnut oil.

Conjugated linoleic acid – full fat milk, cheese- processed, Parmesan, Romano.

PROCESSING LOSSES

Hydrogenation of unsaturated fats during processing destroys a significant proportion of the active components.

Variable loss on exposure to light and heat.

FACTORS INCREASING DEMAND

Alcohol, arthritis, Alzheimer's disease, bile and pancreatic problems, breast feeding, coeliac disease, cystic fibrosis, deficiency in vitamin B6, zinc and magnesium; diabetes, elevated triglycerides and cholesterol, excess saturated fat intake, glaucoma, heart disease, inflammatory disorders, immune disorders, miscarriages, obesity, Parkinson's disease, premature infants, skin disorders, smoking, sterility in males, stress, thirst, trans fatty acid dietary intake.

FUNCTIONS FACILITATED

Blood coagulation, cell to tissue communication, growth, blood triglyceride control (lowers), maintenance of cellular membrane structure and fluidity, modulator of leukotriene synthesis i.e. inflammatory mediator chemicals, prostaglandin precursors, regulates inflammation reactions.

Essential structural component of CNS, facilitates memory, learning and neuronal plasticity.

Omega 3 fatty acids

Increase bleeding time, reduce platelet aggregation and blood viscosity, decrease fibrinogen levels and thrombin formation, down-regulate the genes involved in kainate glutamate receptor expression, increase the adhesion of probiotic bacteria to intestinal wall, increase red blood cell deformability, decrease LDL lipoprotein and triglycerides, regulate inflammatory prostaglandin formation, up regulate cytochrome-C and TNF activity.

Conjugated Linoleic Acid (CLA)

Anticarcinogenic and tumour retardant, anti-inflammatory action, decreases body weight, decreases Bcl2 activity, hypolipidemic, increases lean body mass, promotes apoptosis, reduces insulin resistance, reduces the proliferation of cancer cells, stimulates gene protein p53, stimulates PPAR-alpha.

DEFICIENCY MAY CAUSE OR BE ASSOCIATED WITH:

Acne, blurred vision, ease of bruising, dry, itching, peeling, flaking skin; dry, brittle hair; endocrine dysfunction, decreased EPA/AA ratio in plasma-free fatty acids in angina patients, eye strain with reading, gall stones, headaches, impaired immune response, impaired reproduction, inflammation, kidney damage, nasal problems, neuralgia, pain, paraesthesia, poor wound healing, reproductive failure, respiratory infections, rigid cell membranes, scaly red skin, thirst, varicose veins, visual clouding, xerosis.

THERAPEUTIC USES

Alcoholism, allergy, angina, benign prostatic hyperplasia, hypertriglyceridemia, burns, Crohn's disease, diabetes, elevated blood fats, fat malabsorption, gall bladder disease, heart disease, multiple sclerosis, nephrotic syndrome, skin disorders – acne, eczema, psoriasis, trauma, ulcerative colitis.

GLA – Alcoholism, allergy, atopic eczema, attention deficit disorders, breast pain, depression, diabetes, dry eye syndrome (Sjogren's syndrome), fibrocystic breast disease, glaucoma, high blood cholesterol, hyperactivity, hypertension, obesity, premenstrual syndrome, primary liver cell cancer, Raynaud's syndrome, scleroderma, skin cancer.

DHA/EPA – Atherosclerosis, aggression, Alzheimer's disease, autoimmune disorders, behavioural disturbances, bronchial asthma, cachexia, cancer, chronic fatigue syndrome, chronic inflammation, coronary heart disease, diabetes, forgetfulness, headache, hearing difficulties, hostility, hypertension, to inhibit platelet aggregation, lupus inflammation, multiple sclerosis, muscular degeneration, poor appetite, to reduce angiogenesis, rheumatoid arthritis, thrombosis, tinnitus, viral infection, weakness.

EPA balances the immune system and reduces arachidonic acid levels in cell membranes, reduces PGE2 synthesis.

DHA – Breast feeding, improve brain function, support retinal and spermatozoa function, to aid attention deficit disorder

and Down's syndrome, dyslexia, cystic fibrosis, reduce triglyceride concentrations, depression, to enhance NO production in coronary arteries, infant development.

DHA is involved in neuro-membrane stability and transmission of serotonin, dopamine and nor-adrenalin; which regulate mood and cognitive dysfunction of depression.

CLA – Cancer (breast, colorectal, liver, lung and prostate), diabetes type-2, glioblastoma, hyperlipidemia, leukaemia, melanoma, weight control.

DAILY DOSAGE	
Linoleic acid (w6-EFA) GLA = 1-3gm	5-8% of calories
Linolenic acid (w3-EFA) (6% of alpha linolenic acid is converted to EPA and 3.8% to DHA)	2-4% of calories
DHA/EPA = 1-3gm/day Conjugated linoleic acid (w6-EFA) CLA = 1-4 gm (or 1-1.5% of diet)	

EFFECTS OF OVERDOSAGE AND TOXICITY
>20% of calories increases the demand for vitamin E and other antioxidant nutrients.
May increase the risk of cancer due to excess lipid peroxidation.
May cause temporary thrombocytopenia.

TECHNICAL NOTES

SYNERGISTIC NUTRIENTS

Vitamin A, B_3, B_6, E, bioflavonoids, magnesium, methionine, selenium, quercetin, zinc.

DRUG/NUTRIENT INTERACTIONS

DHA/EPA reduces the toxicity of cyclosporin and lowers the hyperlipidemia associated with etretinates.

STRUCTURE OF GAMMA LINOLEIC ACID (GLA)

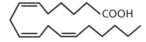

STRUCTURE OF LINOLEIC, LINOLENIC ACID & CONJUGATED LINOLEIC ACID (CLA)

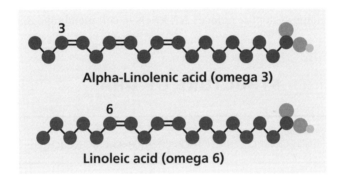

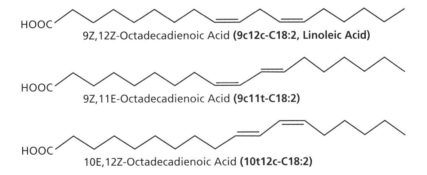

9Z,12Z-Octadecadienoic Acid **(9c12c-C18:2, Linoleic Acid)**

9Z,11E-Octadecadienoic Acid **(9c11t-C18:2)**

10E,12Z-Octadecadienoic Acid **(10t12c-C18:2)**

Conjugated linoleic acid (9c11t-C18:2 and 10t12c-C18:2)

STRUCTURE OF EPA

Eicosapentaenoic acid 20:5n-3	$CH_3CH_2CH=CHCH_2CH=CHCH_2CH=CHCH_2CH=CHCH_2CH=CH(CH_2)_3COOH$
C20 H30 02	

EPA balances the immune system & reduces AA levels in cell membrane & reduces PGE2 synthesis.

STRUCTURE OF DHA

Docosahexaenoic acid 22:6n-3	$CH_3CH_2CH=CHCH_2CH=CHCH_2CH=CHCH_2CH=CHCH_2CH=CHCH_2CH=CH(CH_2)_2COOH$
C22 H32 02	

DHA involved in neuro membrane stability & transmission of serotonin, dopamine & Nor adrenalin, which regulate mood & cognitive dysfunction of depression.

Folic Acid

Folacin, pteroyl-mono-glutamic acid, Vitamin B9

SOURCE
Barley, beans, eggs, endive, green leafy vegetables, lentils, liver, organ meats, sprouts, soybeans, yeast.

PROCESSING LOSSES
Unstable to heat, acid, light.

Storage loss – 20-75%.

Cooking – 65%.

FACTORS INCREASING DEMAND
Ageing, alcoholism, anaemia, antibiotic therapy, anticoagulant therapy, B_{12} deficiency, blood loss, burns, chemically sensitive individuals, coeliac disease, diarrhoea, gastric resection, 5-fluorouracil use, genetic abnormalities, haemodialysis, haemolytic anaemia, Hodgkin's disease, lactation, leukaemia, lung cancer, mental illness, methotrexate, MTHFR polymorphsim, oral contraceptive use, phenytoin, pregnancy, premature and low birth weight infants, retardation.

FUNCTIONS FACILITATED
Coenzyme in purine-pyrimidine metabolism, differentiation of embryonic nervous tissue, DNA repair, growth, NO production (increased), intermediate carrier of one carbon group, maturation of blood cells, metabolism of tyrosine and histidine, methylations, nucleic acid synthesis and metabolism; reduces expression of chromosomal mutations, synthesis of noradrenaline, serotonin, choline.

DEFICIENCY MAY CAUSE OR BE ASSOCIATED WITH:
Anaemia (megaloblastic or microcytic), anorexia, apathy, bronchial metaplasia, cervical dysplasia, cognitive delay, colorectal adenomas, constipation, chromosome breaks, cracks on the lips, diarrhoea, dyskinesia, dyspnoea, fatigue, forgetfulness, glossitis, growth impairment, headaches, hostility, hyperhomocyst(e)inaemia, incorporates uracil into DNA, insomnia, intestinal lesions, irritability, leukopenia, loss of libido, mental sluggishness, myopia, neural tube defects, palpitations, paranoid behaviour, psychomotor retardation, regression, red tongue, reproductive failures, restless legs, seizures, skin disorders, weakness, weight loss.

THERAPEUTIC USES
Acne vulgaris, ADHD, ageing, alcoholism, anaemia, aphthous stomatitis, atherosclerosis, autism, biopterin substitution, cervical dysplasia, Crohn's disease, diabetes (Type II), Down's Syndrome, endothelial dysfunction, fatigue, folate inhibitory drug use, genetic abnormalities, gout, hyperhomocyst(e)inaemia, Lesch-Nyhan disease, lung cancer, memory loss, menstrual problems, mental illness, myopia, neural tubular defects, obesity, patients on epileptic medication, poor libido, pregnancy, premature infants, restenosis, stress, zinc deficiency.

DAILY DOSAGE	
RDA	400 µg
SR	1-5 mg
Infants	100 µg
Children (1-3yrs)	200 µg
Pregnant or nursing mothers	800 µg

EFFECTS OF OVERDOSAGE AND TOXICIT

Essentially non-toxic

>15mg can cause:
Abdominal distension, anorexia, flatulence, hyperactivity, irritability, malaise, nausea, sleep disturbances, vivid dreams.

Muscle restlessness & occasional seizures noted. Large dosage must be accompanied with B_{12}.

TECHNICAL NOTES

SYNERGISTIC NUTRIENTS

Vitamin B_2, B_3, B_5, B_6, B_{12}, C, biopterin, biotin, copper, iron, magnesium, methionine, serine, zinc.

DRUGS/NUTRIENT INTERACTIONS

Decrease folate absorption:
  Antacids – aluminum hydroxide, aluminum carbonate, magnesium carbonate, magnesium hydroxide, magnesium oxide, magnesium trisilicate, aluminum magnesium hydroxide sulfate.
  Bile acid sequestrants – cholestyramine, colestipol, colesevelam
  H2 receptor antagonists – cimetidine, famotidine, nizatidine, ranitidine
  Potassium-sparing diuretics – amiloride, triamterene, spironolactone

Decrease blood or tissue folate levels:
  Alcohol, Anticonvulsants – phenytoin, carbamazepine, primidone, gabapentin, valproic acid, felbamate, lamotrigine, mephenytoin, fosphenytoin, clonazepam, ethosuximide, diazepam, clorazepate dipotassium, levatiracetam, tiagabine, topiramate, methsuximide, phensuximide, trimethadione, magnesium sulfate, acetazolamide, oxcarbazepine, zonisamide, ethotoin.

Corticosteroids – prednisone, hydrocortisone, methylprednisolone, prednisolone, betamethasone, budesonide, triamcinolone, dexamethasone, cortisone, beclomethasone, flunisolide, fluticasone, fludrocortisone, mometasone
Oral contraceptives – norethindrone, ethynodiol diacetate, norgestrel, norgestimate, ethinyl estradiol, drospirenone, desogestrel, levonorgestrel
Metformin, methotrexate

Increase folate urinary secretion:
  Salicylate – Aspirin, choline salicylate, sodium salicylate, magnesium salicylate, salsalate, diflunisal, sodium thiosalicylate

Interrupt folic acid metabolism:
  NSAIDs – ibuprofen, naproxin, etodolac, flurbiprofen, indomethacin, ketorolac tromethamine, mefenamic acid, nabumetone, oxaprozin, sulindac, tolmentin, diclofenac, fenoprofen, ketoprofen, meclofenamate, meloxicam, piroxicam, celecoxib, rofecoxib, valdecoxib
  Trimethoprim containing antibiotics – trimethoprim (TMP), trimethoprim and sulfamethoxazole (TMP-SMZ), trimetrexate glucuronate
  Sulfasalazine

Lower body folic acid levels:
  Aminopterin, Barbiturates, Celecoxib, Cycloserine, Dyazide, Dyrenium, Famotidine, Nizatidine, Pancreatic Enzymes, Phenothiazines, Pyrimethamine, 5-Fluorouracil.

TARGET TISSUES
Bone marrow, kidney, liver, lymph nodes.

ENZYME SYSTEMS INVOLVED
- Activates – reductases (dihydro-folate).
- Coenzyme forms – e.g. folacin, 10-formyl-FH4, 5, 10, methylene-FH4.

- Conjugases – e.g. folic acid conjugase.
- Synthetases – e.g. formyl tetrahydro-folate synthetase.
- Transferases – e.g. serine transhy-droxymethylase, formyl-glutamate formyl transferase.

DEFICIENCY SYMPTOMS AS RELATED TO METABOLIC ACTION	
Anaemia	Decreased synthesis of nucleic acids and porphyrins.
Intestinal disturbances	Indirect relationship with other vitamins.

STRUCTURE OF FOLIC ACID

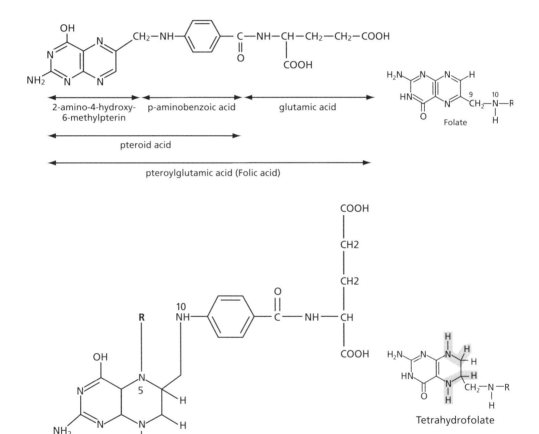

	R	Oxidation state
N5 formyl THFA	-CHO	formate
N10 formyl THFA	-CHO	formate
N5 formimino THFA	-CH=NH	formate
N5,10 methenyl THFA	>CH	formate
N5,10 methylene THFA	>CH2	formaldehyde
N5 methyl THFA	-CH3	methanol

STRUCTURE OF FOLIC ACID (cont)

Folic acid pteroyl-L-glutamic acid, folate or folacin is the dietary precursor to tetrahydro-folate (THF) which plays a key role in a number of different one-carbon transfers such as those involved in purine and pyrimidine synthesis.

The coenzyme forms are actually the reduced products of folic acid. The main function of 5, 6, 7, 8-tetrahydrofolate (THFA) is as a carrier of a C1 (methanoate) unit in the biosynthesis of purines, serines and glycine. The nitrogen atoms at 5 and 10 positions are reactive sites of the molecule.

Vitamin K

Phylloquinone (K1), Menadione (K3), Menaquinone (K2).
Phylloquinone (2-Me-3 phytyl-1-4 napthoquinone) sourced from plants.
Menaquinone (2-Me-3-polyisoprenyl-1-4-napthoquinone) bacterial source.

SOURCE

Bacterial synthesis in the gut, asparagus, broccoli, cabbage, camembert cheese, eggs, kale, kelp, lettuce, liver, oats, pork, soy beans, beef liver, spinach, soybean oil.

Vitamin K1 is found in plants.
Vitamin K2 is synthesized by bacteria in the gut.
Vitamin K3 is converted to K2 by gut bacteria.

PROCESSING LOSSES

Unstable to light or alkali.

FACTORS INCREASING DEMAND

Apo-4 phenotypes, biliary obstruction, blue babies, calcium supplementation, coeliac disease, consumption of irradiated food, Crohn's disease, diarrhoea, extensive surgery, gall and liver disease, high salicylate diet, intestinal infections, long-term parenteral nutrition, mothers in labour, over-dosage with anticoagulants, post menopausal women, rancid fat intake, rheumatoid arthritis, trauma, ulcerative colitis, vitamin A and E excess.

FUNCTIONS FACILITATED

Blood clotting, bone mineralisation, calcium metabolism, synthesis of lung surfactant apo-protein (cofactor), sphingolipid metabolism (cofactor), cofactor of microsomal enzyme glutamyl carboxylase, differentiation of leukemic cells and induces cell apoptosis, growth, improves brain tissue repair, cofactor in plasma proteins C and S, osteocalcin and matrix Gla protein synthesis, prevents neuronal apoptosis, production of hepatic proteins C and S, which prevent clot formation; promotes the breakdown of clots, production of prothrombin, factors II, IX, VII, X. Supports function of pancreatic beta cells.

Increases production of osteocalcin that improves bone calcification & the proliferation of pancreatic beta cells, reduces wrinkle action by preventing calcification of tissues.

Vitamin K2 inhibits microsomal lipid peroxidation and suppresses the deposition of calcium in the aorta i.e. inhibition of arterial calcification as well as skin, thus reducing wrinkling of skin.

DEFICIENCY MAY CAUSE OR BE ASSOCIATED WITH:

Birth defects (underdeveloped nose, mouth and mid face, shortened fingers, cupped ears, flat nasal bridge), bone abnormalities, cognitive impairment, decreased vitality, eye haemorrhage, easy bruising, gastrointestinal bleeding, glucose intolerance, haemorrhages, haematomas, hematuria, hip fracture, hypo-prothrombinaemia, increased clotting time, joint hypermobility, lowered bone density, mitral valve collapse, mucosal bleeding, nose bleeds, osteoporosis, osteopenia, premature ageing.

THERAPEUTIC USES

Acute leukaemia, ageing, Alzheimer's disease, arteriosclerosis, astrocytomas, biliary obstruction, bruising, calcium kidney stones, cerebral haemorrhage, child birth, coeliac disease, colitis, Crohn's disease, cystic fibrosis, diabetes, low bone density, fractures, gliomas, glucose intolerance, poor mitochondrial function; Paget's disease, pain, pancreatic insufficiency, periodontal disease, rheumatoid arthritis, surgery, varicose veins, vitamin D_2 toxicity, anti-wrinkling.

DAILY DOSAGE	
RDA	70-150µg or 1µg per kg weight
SR	2-20 mg
RDA by age:	
0-0.5 yrs	5 µg
0.5-1 yrs	10 µg
1-yrs	15 µg
4-6 yrs	20 µg
7-10 yrs	30 µg
11-14 yrs	45 µg
15-18 yrs	55 µg
Adult <25 yrs	70 µg
Adult >25 yrs	80 µg

Pregnant women taking anti-convulsants should take 20 mg/day for 2 weeks prior to delivery to prevent foetal haemorrhage.

Deficiency state determined by measuring des-γ-carboxy prothrombin (DCP).

EFFECTS OF OVERDOSAGE AND TOXICITY

Porphyrinuria and possible thrombosis, vomiting – mainly with menadione.

- While phylloquinone is non-toxic, menadione can cause toxicity and is the one to be careful with. Menadione can cause: haemolytic anaemia, hyperbilirubinemia and kernicterus, decreased appetite, decreased movement or activity, difficulty in breathing, enlarged liver, general body swelling, irritability, muscle stiffness, paleness, yellow eyes or skin.

TECHNICAL NOTES

SYNERGISTIC NUTRIENTS
Vitamin A, B_3, B_6, C, Calcium, E, C, D, Co enzyme Q_{10}, manganese.

DRUG/NUTRIENT INTERACTIONS

Decrease vitamin K absorption:
  Bile acid sequestrants – cholestyramine, colestipol, colesevelam
  Mineral oil
Decrease gut synthesis of vitamin K:
  Antibiotics – Aminoglycosides, Cephalosporins, Fluoroquinolones, Quinolones, Macrolides, Penicillins, Sulfonamides, Tetracyclines, Trimethoprin-containing antibiotics, Carbapenems, Monobactams, chloramphenicol, spectinomycin, Streptogramins, vancomycin, Oxalodinones, Lincosamides, Nitrofurans
Increase vitamin K breakdown:
  Anticonvulsants – phenytoin, carbamazepine, primidone, gabapentin, valproic acid, felbamate, lamotrigine, mephenytoin, fosphenytoin, clonazepam, ethosuximide, diazepam, clorazepate dipotassium, levatiracetam, tiagabine, topiramate, methsuximide, phensuximide, trimethadione, magnesium sulfate, acetazolamide, oxcarbazepine, zonisamide, ethotoin.
Vitamin K interfering with drug action:
  Coumarin anticoagulants – warfarin
  Anticoagulant medications – heparin, dalteparin, tinzaparin, enoxaparin, danaparoid sodium, antithrombin III, lipirudin, argatroban, bivalirudi.
Decrease vitamin K status or increase demand for vitamin:
  Alcohol, anabolic steroids, butylated hydroxy toluene, Cefamandole, Cefperazone, Phenobarbital, salicylates, sulpha drugs, Tricrynafen, mega doses of Vitamins A & E.

DEFICIENCY SYMPTOMS AS RELATED TO METABOLIC ACTION	
Haemorrhage	Decreased synthesis of prothrombin and other clotting factors by the liver.
Osteoporosis	Decreased calcium bonding by osteocalcin results in increased urinary excretion of calcium.
Calcification of tissue	Gla – a protein that inhibits calcium precipitation
Atheroma	increase precipitation of calcium in atheroma plaques and increase in kidney stone formation.

TARGET TISSUES

Bone, kidney, liver, vascular system, pancreas.

ENZYME SYSTEM INVOLVED

- Vitamin K reductase, oxidative phosphorylation, respiratory chain enzyme involvement.
- Cofactor in carboxylase, which is involved in bone metabolism.

STRUCTURES OF VITAMIN K

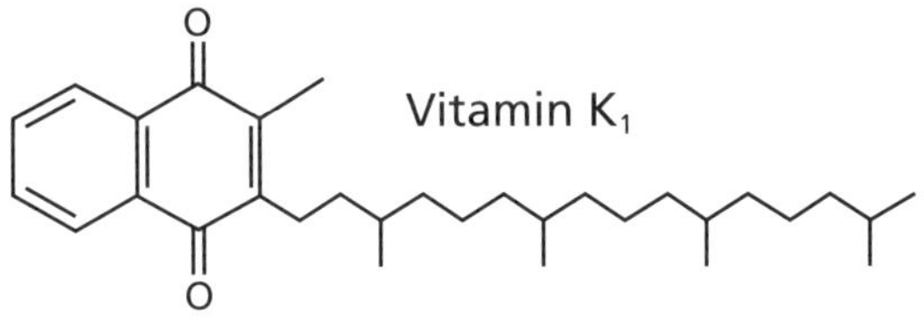

Vitamin K1 or phylloquinone (distributed in liver and heart low in brain tissue)

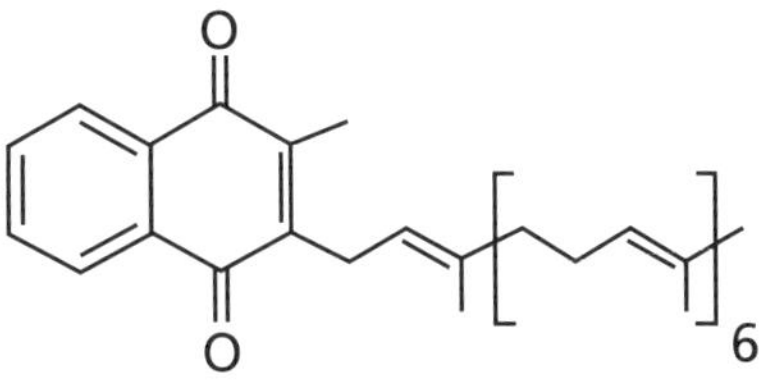

MK-7
Vitamin K2 or Menquinones

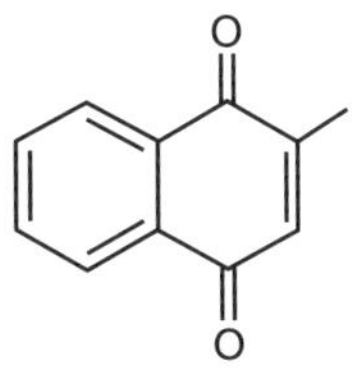

Menadione
Vitamin K3 or Menadione or
2-methyl-1,4-naphthoquinone

Vitamin K2 has a poly-isoprenoid unsaturated side-chain of various length, with isoprene units varying from 4 to 13. These compounds are called menaquinones-n or MK-n. Menaquinones (mainly MK-4) are present at concentrations exceeding those of phylloquinone in pancreas, salivary gland and brain.

CHAPTER 2

Amino Acids

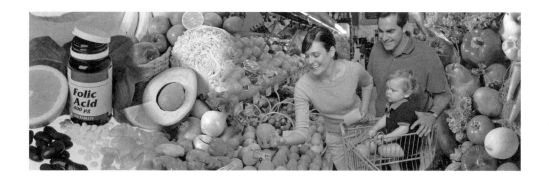

Amino Acids

All amino acids have the same general formula:

$$
\begin{array}{c}
\text{carboxyl end} \\
\text{COO}^- \\
|\\
\text{amino end} \quad \text{H}_3\text{+N} - \text{C} - \text{H} \quad \alpha \text{ carbon}\\
|\\
\text{R}\\
\text{side chain}
\end{array}
$$

The twenty amino acids found in biological systems are:

Amino Acids for Humans		
Non essential	**Essential**	****Conditionally Essential**
Alanine	Histidine (infants)	Arginine
Asparagine	Isoleucine	Cysteine
Aspartate	Leucine	Glycine
Cysteine	Lysine	Glutamine
Glutamate	Methionine	Proline
Glutamine	Phenylalanine	Taurine
Glycine	Threonine	Tyrosine
Proline	Tryptophan	Histidine (adults)
Serine	Valine	Serine (in uremia)
Tyrosine		Tyrosine

** If the body is out of balance or diseased, these amino acids become essential and must be provided from food or supplements.

Amino acids with hydrophobic side groups

Valine (val): COO$^-$, $^+$H$_3$H—C—H, CH, H$_3$C / CH$_3$

Leucine (leu): COO$^-$, $^+$H$_3$H—C—H, CH$_2$, CH, H$_3$C / CH$_3$

Isoleucine (ile): COO$^-$, $^+$H$_3$H—C—H, H—C—CH$_3$, CH$_2$, CH$_3$

Methionine (met): COO$^-$, $^+$H$_3$H—C—H, CH$_2$, CH$_2$, S, CH$_3$

Phenylalanine (phe): COO$^-$, $^+$H$_3$H—C—H, CH$_2$, (benzene ring)

Amino acids with hydrophilic side groups

Asparagine (asn): COO$^-$, $^+$H$_3$H—C—H, CH$_2$, C, H$_3$C / O

Glutamic acid (glu): COO$^-$, $^+$H$_3$H—C—H, CH$_2$, CH$_2$, COO$^-$

Glutamine (gln): COO$^-$, $^+$H$_3$H—C—H, CH$_2$, CH$_2$, C, H$_2$N / O

Histidine (his): COO$^-$, $^+$H$_3$H—C—H, CH$_2$, C—N$^+$H, CH, HC—N, H

Lysine (lys): COO$^-$, $^+$H$_3$H—C—H, CH$_2$, CH$_2$, CH$_2$, CH$_2$, NH$_3^+$

Arginine (arg): COO$^-$, $^+$H$_3$H—C—H, CH$_2$, CH$_2$, CH$_2$, C=NH$_2^+$, NH$_2$

Aspartic acid (asp): COO$^-$, $^+$H$_3$H—C—H, CH$_2$, COO$^-$

Amino acids that are in between

Glycine (gly): COO$^-$, $^+$H$_3$H—C—H, H

Alanine (ala): COO$^-$, $^+$H$_3$H—C—H, CH$_3$

Serine (ser): COO$^-$, $^+$H$_3$H—C—H, C—OH, H

Threonine (thr): COO$^-$, $^+$H$_3$H—C—H, C—OH, CH$_3$

Threonine (thr): COO$^-$, $^+$H$_3$H—C—H, CH$_2$, (benzene ring), OH

Tryptophan (trp): COO$^-$, $^+$H$_3$H—C—H, CH$_2$, C, HC—N, H (indole ring)

Cysteine (cys): COO$^-$, $^+$H$_3$H—C—H, CH$_2$, SH

Proline (pro): COO$^-$, $^+$H$_2$H—C—H, H$_2$C, CH$_2$, CH$_2$, H$_2$

AMINO ACIDS GROUPED BY CHARACTERISTICS

Group Characteristic	Amino Acid Name	Abbreviation
Hydrophobic Non-Polar	Alanine	Ala
	Valine	Val
	Leucine	Leu
	Isoleucine	Ile
	Proline	Pro
	Methionine	Met
	Phenylalanine	Phe
	Tryptophan	Trp
Hydrophilic Polar	Glycine	Gly
	Serine	Ser
	Threonine	Thr
	Cysteine	Cys
	Asparagine	Asn
	Glutamine	Gln
	Tyrosine	Tyr
Hydrophilic Acidic	Aspartic Acid	Asp
	Glutamic Acid	Glu
Hydrophilic Basic	Lysine	Lys
	Arginine	Arg
	Histidine	His

GLYCOGENIC AND/OR KETOGENIC AMINO ACIDS

Glycogenic	Ketogenic	Both Glycogenic and Ketogenic
Alanine	Leucine	Isoleucine
Arginine	Lysine	Phenylalanine
Asparagine		Threonine
Aspartic Acid		Tyrosine
Cysteine		Tryptophan
Glutamic Acid		
Glycine		
Histidine		
Methionine		
Proline		
Serine		

Amino acid	Made from	Degraded to	Glycogenic or Ketogenic	Comments
alanine	pyruvate	pyruvate	glycogenic	large amount in cells
arginine	glutamate	glutamate	glycogenic	strongly basic, urea cycle
asparagine	aspartate	aspartate	glycogenic	glycoproteins
aspartate	Oxalo-acetate	Oxalo-acetate	glycogenic	acidic, large amount in cells
cysteine	methionine*	pyruvate	glycogenic	-SH group
glutamate	Oxo-glutarate	Oxo-glutarate	glycogenic	acidic, very large amount in cells
glutamine	glutamate	glutamate	glycogenic	large amount in cells
glycine	serine	one-carbon pool***	glycogenic	no side chain, collagen
histidine	essential	glutamate	glycogenic	weak base
isoleucine	essential	acetyl-CoA + propionyl-CoA	mixed	branched side-chain
leucine	essential	acetyl-CoA	ketogenic	branched side-chain
lysine	essential	not known	mixed	long side chain, basic
methionine	essential	propionyl-CoA	glycogenic	contains sulphur, methyl donor
phenylalanine	essential	tyrosine	mixed	aromatic, phenylketonuria
proline	glutamate	glutamate	glycogenic	imino acid
serine	Phospho-glycerate	pyruvate	glycogenic	-OH group
threonine	essential	disputed****	glycogenic	-OH group
tryptophan	essential	not known	mixed	aromatic
tyrosine	Phenyl-alanine**	fumarate + aceto-acetate	mixed	aromatic, phenolic
valine	essential	propionyl-CoA	glycogenic	branched side-chain

Notes:
- * Cysteine is conditionally essential – it can be formed from methionine
- ** Tyrosine is conditionally essential – it can be formed from phenylalanine
- *** Multiple pathways for glycine degradation
- **** Multiple pathways for threonine degradation

Amino Acids by Structure

Aliphatic	Alanine
	Glycine
	Isoleucine
	Leucine
	Proline
	Valine
Aromatic	Phenylalanine
	Tryptophan
	Tyrosine
Acidic	Aspartic Acid
	Glutamic Acid
Basic	Arginine
	Histidine
	Lysine
Hydroxylic	Serine
	Threonine
Sulfur-Containing	Cysteine
	Methionine
	Taurine
Amidic (containing amide group)	Asparagine
	Glutamine

Alanine

Alpha amino propionic acid

SOURCE

Most protein sources (composes 7-8% of all proteins), cottage cheese, lactalbumin, legumes, muscle meat, pork, seafood, wheat germ, whey protein.

FACTORS INCREASING DEMAND

Cancer

BODY FUNCTIONS FACILITATED

Activates glucagon release, antiketogenic, contributes to thymus growth, cytoprotective of kidney cells, helps metabolise tryptophan and vitamin B6, increases lymphocyte division, inhibitor of pyruvate kinase, increases synthesis of HSP70 (stress protein), inhibitory neurotransmitter, regulator of glucose metabolism, source of energy for muscle tissue and brain and strengthens immune system by increasing antibody production.

Plays an important part in balancing levels of nitrogen and glucose in the body. It plays an integral part in the glucose-pyruvate, alanine-pyruvate-glucose cycle.

THERAPEUTIC USES

Agitated depression, athletes, cancer, diabetes, enlarged prostate, high cholesterol, hypoglycaemia, insulin dependence, kidney stone prevention, kidney failure, low protein diets, poor immunity, post-exercise ketosis, renal disease.

DAILY DOSAGE	
SR	200-600 mg

TECHNICAL NOTES

SYNERGISTIC NUTRIENTS

Glycine, arginine, aspartate, leucine
Competes with taurine transport.

PHYSICAL PROPERTIES

Non-polar hydrophobic, neutral amino acid, aliphatic.

STRUCTURE OF L- ALANINE

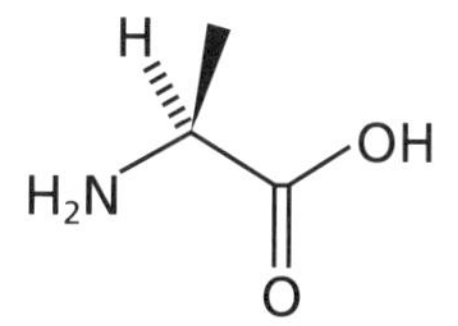

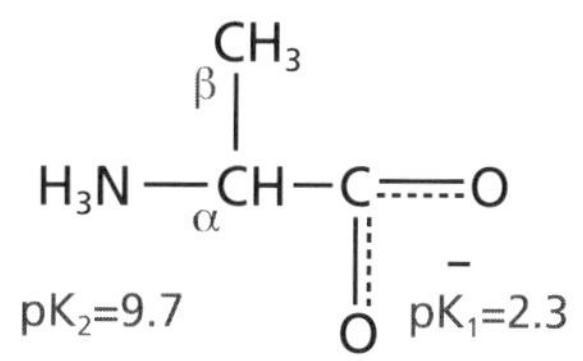

$pK_2=9.7$ $pK_1=2.3$

2-aminopropanoi acid
$C_3H_7NO_2$

2-aminopropanoi acid $C_3H_7NO_2$

Alanine is a hydrophobic molecule. The alpha carbon of alanine is optically active; in proteins, only the L-isomer is found. Alanine and pyruvate are interchangeable by a transamination reaction. It is intimately involved in metabolic pathways such as: glycolysis, gluconeogenesis and citric acid cycle.

Arginine

2-amino – 5-guanidinopentanoic acid

SOURCE

Almonds, beans, carob, cashews, chocolate, dairy products, garlic, ginseng, lactalbumin, peanuts, peanut butter, peas, pecans, raisins, soy protein, sea food, whey, whole wheat.

FACTORS INCREASING DEMAND

Diabetes, high protein diets, infection, injury, intestinal disease, liver failure, lead poisoning, low birth weight infants, poor renal function, pregnancy, sepsis, stress, wounds.

BODY FUNCTIONS FACILITATED

Ammonia detoxification, glycogenesis, methylation; enhances protein synthesis and thymus gland activity; inhibits ornithine decarboxylase, immunomodulator, increases collagen deposition in wounds, increases creatine clearance and glomerular filtration rate, stimulates T lymphocytes; involved in collagen, creatine, creatinine, elastin, glucagon, haemoglobin, increase collagen deposition in wounds, insulin and vasopressin synthesis; precursor of ornithine and urea; precursor for polyamines required for proliferative responses characteristic in healing; metabolised to L-proline – a major constituent of collagen; exerts anti-hypotensive and anti-proliferative effect on vascular smooth muscle; precursor of agmatine, an endogenous non-catecholamine ligand for central alpha 2 adreno receptors (modulates chronic pain sensitivity); improves sperm motility; reduces intra-glomerular pressure (in the kidney) through the production of nitric oxide; reduces toxicity of protein loading; reduces platelet aggregation in hypercholesterolaemia patients; stimulates the immune system by significantly increasing natural killer (NK) and lymphokine activated killer cell cytotoxicity, substrate for the generation of nitric oxide (endothelial relaxing factor); stimulates the release of gastrin, growth hormone and insulin; blocks formation of tumours, stimulates acetyl glutamate synthetise; substrate for the enzymes: arginase, arginine-glycine transaminase, myotrophin synthase, arginine decarboxylase and nitric oxide synthetase; wound healing.

DEFICIENCY MAY CAUSE OR BE ASSOCIATED WITH:

Decreased growth, delayed puberty, fatty liver, glucose intolerance, gut infections, hyper-ammonia, infertility, increases urinary orotate excretion, muscle weakness, skin rashes, trichorrhexis nodosa.

THERAPEUTIC USES

Alcohol abuse, atherosclerosis, balloon angioplasty, burns, cardiac surgery, cancer (35 gm/day diminishes cancer growth and spread), carbon tetrachloride toxicity, chemotherapy, congestive heart failure, chronic pain, diabetes (type2), erection problems, glucose intolerance, gut derived infections, haemodialysis, high blood cholesterol, hyper-ammonia, hypertension (salt sensitive), ischaemic heart disease, intermittent claudication, interstitial cystitis, kidney damage, kidney hypertrophy, liver disease, liver fat metabolism, low birth weight infants, low sperm count, malnutrition, male infertility, muscle building, poor immunity, pre-eclampsia, steroid medication, surgical trauma, sepsis, wound healing, increase collagen deposition in wounds.

SR	1000-6000 mg
Side effects	>2-40gm may cause hyperkalaemia and hyperphosphataemia, a decrease in brain pool of lysine. These result in a loss of appetite, reversible thickening and coarsening of the skin. Increasing dosage due to increased methylation may aggravate schizophrenia.

Green tea extract has a protective affect on arginine-induced toxicity.

(NB. Do not give to patients with herpes or pseudomonas, as it promotes their growth unless lysine is given).

L-arginine may aggravate the effects of cardiac shock.

TECHNICAL NOTES

SYNERGISTIC NUTRIENTS

Aspartic acid, leucine, glycine, lysine, proline, glutamate/glutamine, manganese, methionine, ornithine, vitamin B_6, folic acid, vitamin C, biopterin, citrulline.

The pathways linking arginine, glutamine and proline are bidirectional.

Lysine and ornithine compete with arginine for uptake into the brain.

To increase collagen deposition in wounds-use arginine, leucine & glutamine mixture-14g arginine, 14g glutamine, 3g HMB (Betahydroxy-beta-metlybutyric acid(HMB))

Xylitol can be added as a sweetener to the mixture

Alpha ketoglutarate & ornithine
- Increases arginine, proline & polyamine
- Improves gut morphology & function
- Counteracts trauma-induced poor immunity
- Exerts anabolic effect

PHYSICAL PROPERTIES

Aliphatic, basic amino acid, contingent nutrient (normally synthesised in liver), polar, positively charged.

DRUG/NUTRIENT INTERACTIONS

Potential/Theoretical risk of arginine increasing the effectiveness of a drug – use with caution.

Steroids, cyclosporin A, puromycin amino nucleoside, glyceryl trinitrate.

Amrinone and milrinone, Type III cAMP-dependent phosphodiesterase inhibitors, are additive to L-arginine-dependent vasodilation. Zaprinast and sildenafil, Type V cGMP-dependent phosphodiesterase inhibitors, are synergistic with L-arginine.

L-arginine may potentiate the effects of isosorbide mononitrate and sodium nitroprusside.

Antihypertensive medications – amlodipine, bepridil, diltiazem, felodipine, isradipine, nicardipine, nifedipine, nimodipine,nisoldipine, verapamil, benazepril, captopril, enalapril, lisinopril, fosinopril,moexipril, quinapril, ramipril, trandolapril, perindopril erbumine, atenolol, esmolol, betaxolol, penbutolol, carteolol, bisoprolol, pindolol, metoprolol, timolol, sotalol, acebutolol, nadolol, propranolol, labetalol, carvedilol, methyldopa, clonidine, guanfacine, guanabenz, brimonidine tartrate, dipiprazole, levobunolol,levobetaxolol, metipranolol, reserpine, prazosin, terazosin, doxazosin meylate, guanadrel, guanethidine, isosorbide monohydrate, isosorbide dinitrate, nitroglycerin, hydralazine, minoxidil, papaverine, isoxsuprine, losartan, valsartan, eprosartan mesylate, telmisartan, candesartan cilexetil, irbesartan.

Nitrates – nitroglycerin (various dosage forms), isosorbide mononitrate, isosorbide dinitrate, amyl nitrate.

Sildenafil

Intravenous arginine infusions can cause hyperkalemia, thus drugs that may increase potassium levels should not be taken with this nutrient eg.

Potassium-sparing diuretics – amiloride, triamterene, spironolactone

ACE inhibitors – benazepril, captopril, enalapril, lisinopril, fosinopril, moexipril quinapril, ramipril, trandolapril, perindopril erbumine.

NUTRIENT/NUTRIENT INTERACTIONS

Lysine competes with arginine for cellular uptake.

TARGET TISSUE

Intestine, kidney.

INBORN ERRORS OF METABOLISM

Arginase deficiency	Gives rise to high blood levels of arginine.
Symptoms of:	Mental retardation, spastic diplegia, convulsions. Lysine and ornithine supplementation may be of benefit in these cases.

STRUCTURE OF L-ARGININE

2-amino-5-(diaminomethylideneamino) pentanoic acid $C_6H_{14}N_4O_2$

Arginine has a positively charged guanidino group. Arginine can bind the phosphate anion, and is often found in the active centers of proteins that bind phosphorylated substrates. As a cation, arginine, as well as lysine, plays a role in maintaining the overall charge balance of a protein.

Aspartic Acid

2 amino butanedioic acid, Aspartate, Asparagine

SOURCE

Asparagus, avocado, beans, brown rice, dairy products, eggs, fish, legumes, luncheon meats, NutraSweet, oat flakes, sausage meat, sprouting seeds, whey protein, wild game.

FACTORS INCREASING DEMAND

Stress, opiate withdrawal.

FUNCTIONS FACILITATED

Ammonia detoxification, bone calcification, brain energy metabolism, excitatory neurotransmitter in spinal chord, gluconeogenesis, improves glycolysis in damaged tissue, improves fatty acid oxidation, glycoprotein synthesis, pyrimidine synthesis, transamination and deamination reactions involved in the urea cycle.

Moves NADH from the cytoplasm into the mitochondria to produce ATP.

RELATIVE DEFICIENCY SYMPTOMS

Depression, fatigue, increased serum ammonia levels.

THERAPEUTIC USES

Athletes, bone formation, cardiac surgery, chronic fatigue, helps eliminate toxins; hepatic encephalopathy, hyperammonemia, coronary artery blockage; enhances potassium and magnesium uptake in salt form e.g. magnesium and potassium aspartate.

Potassium aspartate is helpful in treating heart attacks, hypertension and preventing irregular rhythms, and in radiation therapy.

Magnesium aspartate

Stress, cardiac failure, hypertension, poor concentration, pregnancy, hypercholestremia, opiate addiction, cyclosporine induced hypertension and nephrotoxicity.

DAILY DOSAGE	
SR	1.5-2 gm/day

TOXICITY

Similar to monosodium glutamate.

Magnesium and zinc decrease toxicity.

TECHNICAL NOTES

SYNERGISTIC NUTRIENTS

Arginine, citrulline, glutamine, glutamic acid, magnesium, potassium, vitamin B_6, glycine, L-ornithine–L-aspartate (OA).

Glycine acts as a modulator of excitatory aspartic acid neurotransmission in the spinal cord.

PHYSICAL PROPERTIES

Acidic hydrophilic amino acid (polar), aliphatic, negatively charged.

STRUCTURE OF L – ASPARTIC ACID OR ASPARTATE

2-aminobutanedioic acid $C_4H_7NO_4$

Aspartic acid is one of two acidic amino acids. Aspartic acid and glutamic acid play important roles as general acids in enzyme active centers, as well as in maintaining the solubility and ionic character of proteins.

Aspartic acid and oxaloacetate are interconvertable by a simple transamination reaction.

Asparagine

(Non essential amino acid)

SOURCE

Asparagus, milk, soy, eggs, fish, meat.

FUNCTIONS FACILITATED

Required precursor for the synthesis of RNA, DNA and ATP, involved in antibody and collagen assembly, cell to cell recognition, precursor of aspartate. Increases oxidative metabolism.

Participates in the metabolic control of cell functions in the brain and nervous system.

DEFICIENCY MAY BE ASSOCIATED WITH:

Autoimmunity, immune system stress, infection and severe allergies.

THERAPEUTIC USES

Infection or sepsis. Diet supplementation with cysteine, threonine, serine, aspartate-asparagine and arginine supports the synthesis of vital proteins to spare body protein catabolism during infection. Reduces fatigue during exercise performed above anaerobic threshold.

SIDE EFFECTS

May increase epileptogenesis

PHYSICAL PROPERTIES

Amide-form of aspartic acid and polar amino acid, water soluble, but electrically neutral.

STRUCTURE OF ASPARAGINE

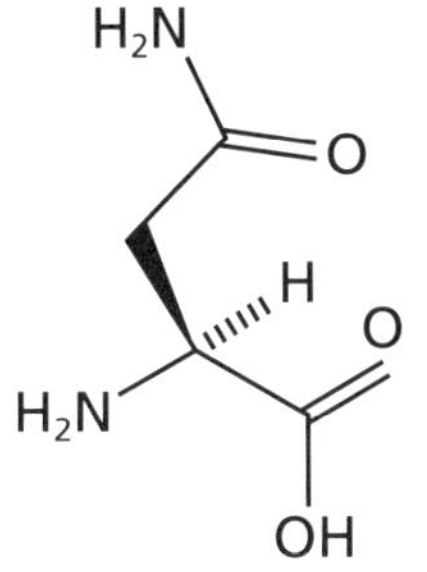

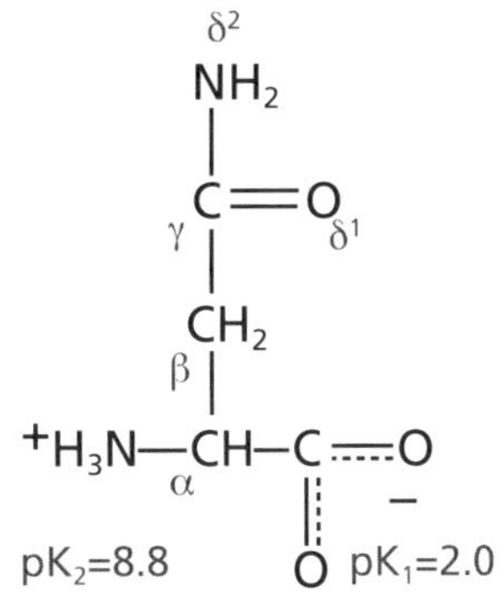

2-amino-3-carbamoyl-propanoic acid $C_4H_8N2O_3$

Asparagine is the amide of aspartic acid. The amide is easily hydrolyzed, converting asparagine to aspartic acid.

Asparagine has a high propensity to hydrogen bonding, since the amide group can accept two and donate two hydrogen bonds. It is found on the surface as well as buried within proteins.

Asparagine is a common site for attachment of carbohydrates in glycoproteins.

Cysteine

2 – amino – 3 mercapto propanoic acid

SOURCE

Beans, beef, brewer's yeast, chicken, cottage cheese, eggs, fish, garlic, liver, milk, sardines, sea food, whey protein.

FACTORS INCREASING DEMAND

Aspirin intake, acetaminophen overdose, alcohol, chemotherapy, cigarette smoking, diabetes, malabsorption syndrome.

FUNCTIONS FACILITATED

Required for the synthesis of insulin, skin, hair, coenzyme A, heparin, biotin, lipoic acid, glutathione, glucose tolerance factor, metallothionein and sulphates; detoxifies chemicals, involved in conjugation reactions, involved in the synthesis of lipoic acid, antioxidant properties.

N-acetylcysteine has been found to reduce the invasiveness and metastatic potential of melanoma cells, and to inhibit endothelial cell invasion by a direct inhibition of matrix metalloproteinases (MMPs); an amino acid transporter across membranes, precursor of taurine, protects stomach and intestinal lining, provides cell protection against radiation and pollution, helps cross-link proteins, aids in bile secretion.

DEFICIENCY MAY BE ASSOCIATED WITH:

Abnormal immune function, cancer, decrease in glutathione synthesis, decrease in sulphation reactions, decreased ability to metabolise drugs and toxic chemicals, poor wound healing, poor skin integrity, psoriasis, psychosis.

High intakes of serine and alanine decrease liver uptake of cysteine.

Cystine

Dimer of two cysteine molecules

THERAPEUTIC USES

Acetaminophen overdose, ageing, AIDS, allergies, asthma, bronchitis, burns, chemical sensitivity, chemotherapy, chronic liver disease, chronic obstructive airway disease, cuts, cyclophosphamide toxicity, cystic fibrosis, cytotoxic effects of chemotherapy, diabetes, doxorubicin toxicity, emphysema, hair weakness and hair loss, heavy metal toxicity, HIV infection, induced liver toxicity, inflammatory conditions, irradiation, sepsis, smokers, psoriasis, virally induced nutritional deficiency, Wilson's disease.

DAILY DOSAGE	
RDA	500 mg/day
SR	200-1500 mg – must be taken with vitamin B6 and C.

Note: L-cysteine supplementation should be accompanied by at least six to eight glasses of water daily in order to prevent cystine renal stones. Some studies indicate that an intake of 3 to 5 grams daily of vitamin C may prevent cystine stones.

TECHNICAL NOTES

SYNERGISTIC NUTRIENTS

Vitamin B_2, B_3, B_6, B_{12}, C, chromium, folic acid, glycine, glutamine, methionine, serine, zinc, selenium, lipoic acid.

DISEASES LINKED WITH AMINO ACID	
Homocystinuria	Deficiency of cystathionine synthetase.
Symptoms	Atherosclerosis, light complexion, failure to thrive, mental retardation.
Treatment	If diet is low in methionine and cystine, supplement with vitamin B_6 (>100 mg), folic acid, vitamin B_{12} and serine

Target Tissues

Liver, brain, kidney, intestine.

Cysteine is predominantly inside cells where its disulphide form cystine is predominantly outside the cell.

Cysteine is taken up 10 times faster than cystine.

PHYSICAL PROPERTIES

Aliphatic, neutral, hydrophilic amino acid, water-soluble.

Cysteine is readily autoxidised to cystine in the extracellular fluid. Once inside the cell, cystine is readily reduced to cysteine.

STRUCTURE OF L- CYSTEINE

2-amino-3-sulfanyl-propanoic acid $C_3H_7NO_2S$

Cysteine is one of two sulfur-containing amino acids; the other is methionine.

Cysteine plays a key role in stabilizing extracellular proteins. Cysteine can react with itself to form an oxidized dimer (Cystine) by formation of a disulfide bond. The environment within a cell is too strongly reducing for disulfides to form, but in the extracellular environment, disulfides can form and play a key role in stabilizing many proteins, such as the digestive enzymes of the small intestine and insulin.

Glutamine & Glutamic Acid

SOURCE

Beans, cottage cheese, dairy products, ham, legumes, sausage meat, most protein sources, ricotta cheese, rolled oats, whey protein.

FACTORS INCREASING DEMAND

Alcoholics (glutamine), burns, critically ill patients, glucocorticoid medication, infection, major surgery, sepsis, shock, stress, tissue injury.

FUNCTIONS FACILITATED

Glutamine

Ammonia detoxification, bone calcification, catalyst for the formation of acetylcholine, conjugation reactions, constituent of glutathione and glucose tolerance factor, controls acid-base balance (renal ammoniagenesis), enhances lymphocyte mitogenic function, essential precursor of nucleotide synthesis, involved in DNA synthesis, fuel for intestinal enterocytes, lymphocytes, macrophages, endothelial cells and renal tubular cells; gastrointestinal support, immune enhancer, improves gut IgA levels, improves gut immunity, L-arginine-NO-metabolism, maintains acid base balance, maintains muscle mass, precursor to gamma amino butyric acid (GABA), gamma hydroxy butyric acid (GHBA) and gamma butyrolactone which act as neuro-inhibitory transmitters; nitrogen transport, promotes healing and bowel rescue, regulates acid/base balance, replenishes amino acid stores, substrate for energy production in hypoxic, anoxic, and dysoxic tissues; shuttle for glutamate (CNS), supports gut mucosal growth, supports renal ammonia genesis, transamination reactions.

Glutamine is the nitrogen donor, involved in the biosynthesis of purines and pyrimidines.

Glutamic acid

Excitatory neurotransmitter, binds to NMDA receptors, involved in memory and learning, mediates neuronal apoptosis through excitotoxicity, associated with ischaemic stroke, epilepsy and Alzheimer's disease; associated with umani taste sensation.

95% of glutamate is metabolised by the gut in the first pass.

Glutamic acid does not cross the blood brain barrier.

DEFICIENCY MAY BE ASSOCIATED WITH

Depression, diarrhoea, leaky gut syndrome, muscle wasting, poor immunity, poor gut immunity, villi atrophy.

THERAPEUTIC USES

Glutamine

Abdominal surgery, ageing, AIDS, alcoholism, autism, behavioural problems, bone formation, chemically sensitive individuals, chemotherapy, CNS nitrogen depletion, depression, epilepsy, exercise trauma, gut irritation, hypertension, immunosuppression, improves IQ, infection, inhibited neurotransmission, irritable bowel syndrome, leaky gut syndrome, physical trauma, poor concentration, radiation damage, radio-chemotherapy, rheumatoid arthritis, senility, sepsis, surgical stress, ulcers, viral induced nutrient deficiency, wound healing.

DAILY DOSAGE		
SR	(Glutamine)	500-30000 mg (20g/Day in TPN Solution)
	Athletes	8-10 g/day
	Trauma	10-30 g/day

EFFECTS OF OVERDOSAGE AND TOXICITY

Excess – Monosodium glutamate (taste enhancer) may give rise to Chinese restaurant syndrome – burning sensation on lips, flushing.

Vitamin B_6 overcomes these symptoms.

Greater than 300 mg of **glutamic acid** may cause mania in some individuals.

Glutamine supplementation is contraindicated in hyper-ammonaemia, ammonia intoxication or nitrogen excess.

TECHNICAL NOTES

SYNERGISTIC NUTRIENTS

Arginine, aspartic acid, folic acid, glucose tolerance factor, glycine, magnesium, manganese, potassium, proline, taurine, vitamin B_6, zinc.

Alpha-keto glutarate has a sparing effect on glutamine pools.

DRUG/NUTRIENT INTERACTIONS

Methotrexate – L-glutamine decreases the elimination of methotrexate from the body.

PHYSICAL PROPERTIES

Glutamate – acidic hydrophilic amino acid (polar), aliphatic, negatively charged.

Glutamine – polar, water soluble, aliphatic, charged molecule.

INBORN ERRORS

Errors in glutamate metabolism involve the inability to join the amino acids cysteine and glycine with glutamate to form glutathione.

TARGET TISSUES

Whole blood, skeletal muscle.

STRUCTURE OF L-GLUTAMIC ACID

$pK_R=4.3$

2-aminopentanedioic acid $C_5H_9NO_4$

Glutamic acid and α-ketoglutarate, an intermediate in the Krebs cycle, are inter-convertible by transamination. Glutamic acid can enter the Krebs cycle for energy metabolism, and be converted by the enzyme glutamine synthetase into glutamine, which is one of the key players in nitrogen metabolism.

Glutamic acid can be easily converted into proline.

STRUCTURE OF L-GLUTAMINE

2-amino-4-carbamoyl-butanoic acid $C_5H_{10}N_2O_3$

Glutamine is the amide of glutamic acid, and is uncharged under all biological conditions.

Glycine

α amino acetate

SOURCE

Gelatine and most protein sources – beans, brewer's yeast, eggs, fish, lactalbumin, sea food, nuts, whey protein.

FACTORS INCREASING DEMAND

Arthritis, cancer, endotoxaemia, high salicylate diet, high urinary hippurate, inflammation, foods rich in benzoic acid – pickles, cranberry, lunch meats.

FUNCTIONS FACILITATED

This amino acid performs the most biochemical functions of any amino acid.

Constituent of collagen, glutathione and many protein hormones; co-agonist with glutamate on the NMDA receptor, down-regulates NADPH oxidase activity, glycogenic, increases growth hormone release, increases renal clearance of uric acid, inhibitory neurotransmitter (activates glycine gated chloride channel), increases stress protein HSP70 production, involved in the synthesis of nucleic acids, bile salts, creatine, haemoglobin and serine; liver detoxification, detoxifies phenols, salicylates, benzoic acid and methionine; lowers triglycerides, reduces residual volume in bladder, modulates the activity of hepatic and alveolar macrophages, neutrophils and lymphocytes; anti-angiogenic effects, anti inflammatory, immunomodulator, cyto-protective, activates chloride channels in plasma membranes, stabilizes protein structures eg cytochrome C, myoglobulin and haemoglobin.

Involved in bile synthesis, improves memory retreival.

THERAPEUTIC USES

Alcoholic hepatitis, arthritis, athletic performance, autoimmune disorder, autoimmune induced tumours, atherosclerosis, benign prostatic hypertrophy, bile synthesis, cancer, CNS trauma, chemical sensitivity, chemically induced ulcers, cyclosporin toxicity, cyclosporine renal injury, detoxification of benzoic acid and salicylates, fatigue, endotoxaemia, epilepsy, gout, haemorrhagic stroke, hypermania, hypoxia, ischaemic reperfusion injury, isovaleric acidaemia, kidney failure, leg ulcers, inflammatory disease, liver transplants, liver ischaemic reperfusion injury, melanoma, memory retrieval, metastasis, myasthenia, nail growth, neurotoxic cell death, poor digestion, prevents cancer spread, respiratory distress syndrome, schizophrenia (improves medication response) sepsis, seizures, spasticity, spinal injuries, stress induced ulcers, stroke, wound healing (in the presence of arginine).

DAILY DOSAGE	
SR	4-30gm/day 200mg/kg/day

EFFECTS OF OVERDOSAGE AND TOXICITY
8 g/kg body weight – hyperexcitability.

TECHNICAL NOTES

SYNERGISTIC NUTRIENTS

Vitamin B_2, B_6, arginine, folic acid, cysteine, serine, threonine, glutamate, aspartate, leucine, taurine.

SOURCES IN THE BODY

Muscle, skin, connective tissue

CONTRA INDICATIONS

For patients with non-ketotic hyperglycaemia:

– Glycine in this condition increases
oxidant stress

– Counteracted by using melatonin,
vitamin E & glutathione

DISEASES LINKED WITH AMINO ACID	
Glycinemia (ketogenic form):	Defect in the enzyme propionyl CoA carboxylase.
Glycinuria	Defect in renal absorption of glycine.
Primary hyperoxaluria	Glycine may be metabolised through the oxalate pathway.

PHYSICAL PROPERTIES

Non polar hydrophobic, neutral amino
acid, water insoluble.

STRUCTURE OF L-GLYCINE

Amino ethanoic acid $C_2H_5NO_2$

Glycine is the smallest of the amino acids.
In aqueous solution at or near neutral pH,
glycine will exist predominantly as the
zwitterion.

Histidine

2-amino – 3 (4-imidazolyl) propanoic acid

SOURCE
Banana, chicken, cottage cheese, egg, fish, meat, legumes, whey protein, wheat germ.

FACTORS INCREASING DEMAND
Alcohol, arthritic conditions, chronic illness, growth, low birth weight infants, post-surgery, uraemic patients.

FUNCTIONS FACILITATED
Chelates copper and zinc, gastric secretion, glycogenesis, improves zinc absorption, increases zinc uptake by brain, increases the release of ACTH during acute stress, involved in the synthesis of collagen, haemoglobin, histamine, myelin sheath, purine, pyrimidine; potentiates the action of TSH-RF and luteinizing hormone releasing factors (LHRF), precursor of histamine (neuro-inhibitor), carnosine and anserine; regulates the release of catecholamines in the hypothalamus and heart, vasodilatory and hypotensive action.

Improves sexual pleasure (with vitamin B_3 and B_6).

DEFICIENCY MAY CAUSE OR BE ASSOCIATED WITH:
Agitation, confusion, decreased food and water intake, decrease in haematocrit, malaise, memory loss, nausea, negative nitrogen balance, nerve deafness, poor hearing, sexual frigidity, skin eruptions.

THERAPEUTIC USES
Allergic conditions, AIDS, anaemia, arthritis, auditory dysfunction, free floating anxiety, heavy metal toxicity, helps improve protein digestion, histopenic schizophrenia, hypertension, inflammation, kidney failure, Parkinson's disease, poor memory, poor stomach acidity, radiation therapy, rheumatoid arthritis, thyroid problems, ulcers, uraemia.

DAILY DOSAGE		
RDA	**Infants** 33 mg/gm body weight	
	Adult 8-10 mg/kg body weight	
SR	Average intake 1-6 gm/day	

TECHNICAL NOTES

SYNERGISTIC NUTRIENTS
Vitamin B_3, B_6, C, biotin, carnosine, calcium, folic acid, linoleic and linolenic acid, manganese, zinc.

(Copper and methionine lower blood histamine levels).

A combination of zinc, histidine and GLA acts as a powerful anti-inflammatory formula.

Histidine 500mg before meals with betaine hydrochloride improves protein digestion.

DISEASES LINKED WITH AMINO ACID	
Histidinaemia	Deficiency in the enzyme histidine alpha deaminase.
Symptoms	Mental retardation, speech defects.

ADVERSE EFFECTS AND TOXICITY
Headache, weakness, drowsiness, nausea, anorexia, painful eyes, changed visual acuity, mental confusion, poor memory, and depression, mental disorders.

Dosages greater than 5% of diet may result in growth depression and a 10-fold increase in brain histidine levels. The levels of isoleucine, leucine, tyrosine, and phenylalanine may decrease in the brain by 50%.

Histidine complexes with copper and may give rise to copper deficiency and hyper- lipidemia. Supplementing with copper, folic acid, methionine and retinol reduces toxicity.

PHYSICAL PROPERTIES

Basic hydrophilic essential amino acid, polar, positively charged, water-soluble.

STRUCTURE OF L-HISTIDINE

2-amino-3-(3H-imidazol-4-yl) propanoic acid $C_6H_9N_3O_2$

Histidine has as a positively charged imidazole functional group.

The imidazole group allows histidine to pay a role in many catalytic reactions. The unprotonated imidazole is nucleophilic and can serve as a general base, while the protonated form can serve as a general acid. The residue can also serve a role in stabilizing the folded structures of proteins.

Isoleucine

2-amino – 3-methyl pentanoic acid

SOURCE

Almonds, beef, chicken, egg, fish, legumes, milk, nuts, pumpkin seeds, soybeans, whey protein.

Animal protein contains on average 42 mg/gm of protein.

FACTORS INCREASING DEMAND

Athletes, liver disease, pre-term infants, renal patients.

FUNCTIONS FACILITATED

Muscle development and repair, essential for the synthesis of dispensable amino acids, glucogenic and ketogenic amino acid, a common component of proteins, peptides and hormones; helps maintain structure of globulin proteins (beta structures), increases glucose uptake by muscles, lowers blood glucose levels, prevents muscle breakdown at high altitudes, prolongs endurance.

Competes with aromatic amino acids for uptake by the brain.

Encourages clotting at site of injury.

DEFICIENCY MAY CAUSE OR BE ASSOCIATED WITH:

Ammonia genesis, ureagenesis, diabetes, EAA excitotoxicity, negative nitrogen balance, poor growth, spasticity, tremors, twitching of muscle extremities, increased portal NH_3 and amino acids, impaired DNA synthesis, catabolism (headaches, dizziness, fatigue and depression; all due to low blood sugar), irritability.

THERAPEUTIC USES

Anorexia nervosa, athletes, heavy exercise, hepatic failure, hyper-ammonia, hypercatabolic states, hyperglycaemia, hypoxia, low birth weight infants, muscle weakness, renal failure, schizophrenia (B_3 dependent type), sepsis, stress, surgery, uraemia, upper gastrointestinal bleeding.

DAILY DOSAGE		
RDA	**Infants** 80 mg/kg body weight	
	Child 28 mg/kg body weight	
	Adult 12 mg/kg body weight	
SR	Average intake 5-10 gm/day	

EFFECTS OF OVERDOSAGE AND TOXICITY

Large dosage may compete with aromatic amino acid transporters across the blood brain barrier resulting in decreased uptake of tryptophan, tyrosine and phenylalanine. This may result in decreased neurotransmitter synthesis (serotonin, dopamine and nor adrenalin) giving rise to depression.

TECHNICAL NOTES

SYNERGISTIC NUTRIENTS

Vitamin B_1, B_3, B_{12}, biotin, folic acid, magnesium.

NUTRIENT/NUTRIENT INTERACTIONS

Phenylalanine, tryptophan, tyrosine – compete with Leucine, isoleucine and valine for transport into the brain.

PHYSICAL PROPERTIES

Non polar hydrophobic, essential branch chain amino acid, aliphatic, water insoluble.

STRUCTURE OF L-ISOLEUCINE

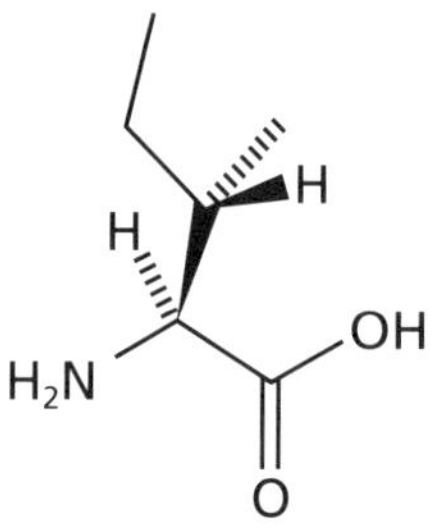

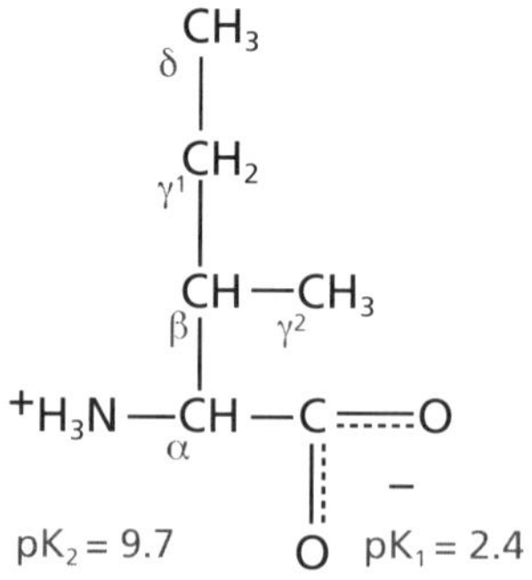

$$CH_3 \quad (\delta)$$
$$|$$
$$CH_2 \quad (\gamma^1)$$
$$|$$
$$CH - CH_3 \quad (\beta) \; (\gamma^2)$$
$$|$$
$$^+H_3N - CH - C \!=\!=\! O \quad (\alpha)$$
$$|$$
$$pK_2 = 9.7 \qquad O \quad pK_1 = 2.4$$

2-amino-3-methylpentanoic acid $C_6H_{13}NO_2$

Isoleucine is one of the three amino acids having branched hydrocarbon side chains. It is usually interchangeable with leucine and occasionally with valine in proteins.

The side chains of these amino acids are not reactive and therefore not involved in any covalent chemistry in enzyme active centres but are critically important for ligand binding to proteins, and therefore, play central roles in protein stability.

Leucine

2-amino – 4-methylpentanoic acid

SOURCE

Almonds, baked beans, beef, cashews, chicken, corn, eggs, fish, lentils, legumes, liver, sea food, soybeans, whey protein, whole wheat.

Animal protein contains on average 70 mg/gm of protein.

FACTORS INCREASING DEMAND

Infants, liver disease, poor digestion, puberty spurts, renal patients, surgery.

BODY FUNCTIONS FACILITATED

Activates glutamate dehydrogenase, competes with aromatic amino acids for brain uptake, component of elastin and protein hormones (enkephalin), growth, enhances skeletal muscle recovery after exercise, essential for the synthesis of dispensable amino acids, helps maintain structure of globulin proteins (alpha structures), increases incorporation of glucose into glycogen, lowers brain levels of serotonin and dopamine, promotes wound healing, reduces appetite, regulates muscle protein synthesis and blood sugar levels, regulates the synthesis of the brain neurotransmitter glutamate, stimulates insulin release, synthesis of leucopeptin – a lysosomal proteinase inhibitor of lipofuscin.

Helps burn visceral fat, regulates blood sugar.

DEFICIENCY MAY CAUSE OR BE ASSOCIATED WITH:

Negative nitrogen balance, poor growth.

Hypoglycaemic symptoms include: dizziness, fatigue, headaches.

THERAPEUTIC USES

Aged individuals, athletic endurance, biliary atresia, body builders, diabetes, dystonia, fatigue, fasting, fever below 101°F, glutamate excitotoxicity, hepatitis, hepatic cirrhosis, hypercatabolic states, hyperglycaemia, kidney failure, liver failure, low birth weight infants, muscle weakness, muscle wasting in the aged, pancreatic dysfunction, Parkinson's disease with olivoponto cerebellar atrophy, stress, surgery, tardive dyskinesia, uraemia, wound healing.

D-leucine may also be used for the treatment of chronic pain.

DAILY DOSAGE		
RDA	Infants	135 mg/kg body weight
	Child	42 mg/kg body weight
	Adult	6-10 mg/kg body weight
SR	Average intake 170-3000 mg/day	

EFFECTS OF OVERDOSAGE AND TOXICITY
Excess (>150mg/kg/body weight) may precipitate pellagra in marginal vitamin B_3 deficiency resulting in neurological symptoms.
Large dosage may compete with aromatic amino acid transporters across the blood brain barrier resulting in decreased uptake of tryptophan, tyrosine and phenylalanine. This may result in decreased neurotransmitter synthesis (serotonin, dopamine and nor adrenalin) giving rise to depression.

TECHNICAL NOTES

SYNERGISTIC NUTRIENTS

Vitamin B_1, B_3, B_6, magnesium, methionine, isoleucine, valine.

NUTRIENT/NUTRIENT INTERACTIONS

Phenylalanine, tryptophan, tyrosine
– compete with Leucine, isoleucine and valine for transport into the brain.

ENZYME SYSTEMS INVOLVED

- D-isomer inhibits neural enkephalinase.

- Leucine inhibits kynurinase, activates picolinate carboxylase.

DISEASES LINKED TO AMINO ACID

Leucine increases B_3 loss in urine.

Leucine intolerance – unknown cause, gives rise to hypoglycaemia.

PHYSICAL PROPERTIES

Non polar hydrophobic essential amino acid, insoluble in water.

Branch chain amino acid, Ketogenic.

STRUCTURE OF L-LEUCINE

2-amino-4-methyl-pentanoic acid $C_6H_{13}NO_2$

Leucine is an amino acid with a branched hydrocarbon side chain. Being hydrophobic it is generally buried in folded proteins.

Lysine

SOURCE

Brewer's yeast, chicken, dairy products, fish, lamb, legumes, lentils, milk, mung bean sprouts, oat flakes, soy bean, water crest, whey protein.

High quality protein contains on average 50 mg/gm of protein.

FACTORS INCREASING DEMAND

Arginine and ornithine supplementation, cancer, excessive exercise, herpes infections, hypothyroidism, low protein diets, macrobiotic diets, protein calorie malnutrition, surgery.

FUNCTIONS FACILITATED

Antiviral activity, binds apoprotein(a), carnitine synthesis, connecting linkage for vitamin B_6 on enzymes, constituent of collagen and elastin, decreases apo(a), decreases iNOS activity during endotoxic shock, increases intestinal absorption of calcium, involved in carnitine synthesis, maintains lean body mass, promotes bone growth, important component of hormonal proteins, precursor of citrulline, prevents glycol-oxidation, promotes both collagen and muscle protein synthesis.

DEFICIENCY MAY CAUSE OR BE ASSOCIATED WITH:

Anaemia, decreased growth, dizziness, endotoxemia, fatigue, fatty acid metabolism problems, inability to concentrate, infertility, irritability, loss of appetite, loss of body weight, loss of bone calcium, loss of sperm motility, nausea, poor immune function, slow growth, tiredness.

THERAPEUTIC USES

Angina, athletic performance, atheroma, arginine excess, Bell's palsy, cancer, cataracts, cold sores, conjunctivitis, cranial nerve pain (associated with herpes), diabetes, female hair loss, herpes infection, hyperglycaemia, infertility, irritable bowel syndrome, lead toxicity, ligament damage, lysinuric protein intolerance, marasmus, Meniere's disease, osteoporosis, stimulator of growth, shingles, spinal injuries, stress, surgery, wound healing.

DAILY DOSAGE		
RDA	**Infants**	99 mg/kg body weight
	Child	44 mg/kg body weight
	Adult	32 mg/kg body weight
SR	Average intake 300-3000 mg/day	

EFFECTS OF OVERDOSAGE AND TOXICITY
>10-15 g/day may cause gastrointestinal upset, including nausea, abdominal cramps, and diarrhoea.
Increase triglycerides and cholesterol levels at high dosage. This may be decreased by supplementing with arginine.

TECHNICAL NOTES

Lysine competes with arginine for transport into the cell.

SYNERGISTIC NUTRIENTS

Vitamin B_2, B_3, B_6, C, bioflavonoids, copper, glutamic acid, iron, methionine, proline, arginine, green tea extract, carnitine.

PHYSICAL PROPERTIES

Basic hydrophilic (polar), essential amino acid, water soluble, positively charged, aliphatic.

Ketogenic amino acid.

DRUG/NUTRIENT INTERACTIONS

Lysine may increase toxicity to gentamycin, neomycin and streptomycin.

STRUCTURE OF L-LYSINE

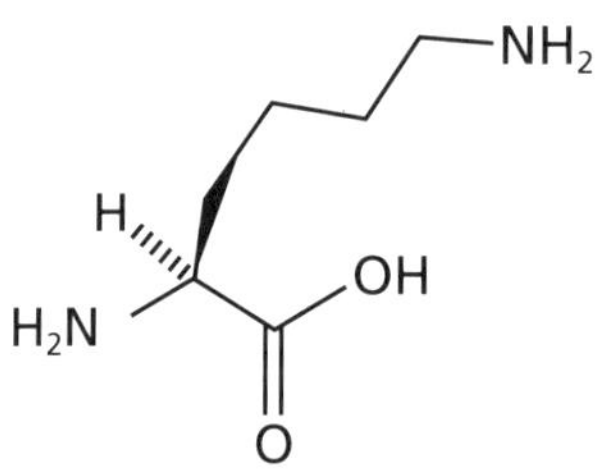
NH2
H
H2N
OH
O

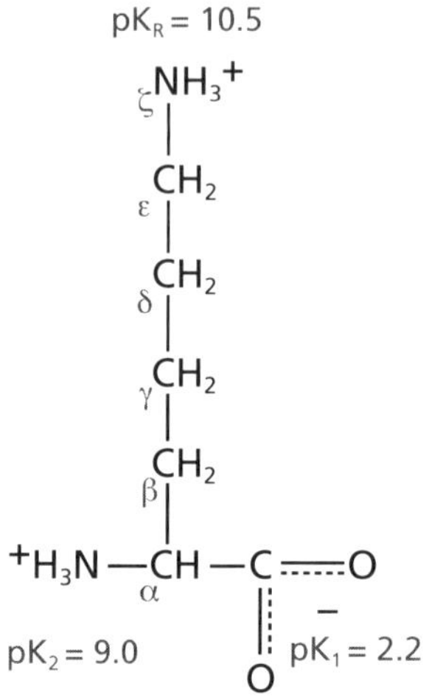
pKR = 10.5
NH3+
ζ
CH2
ε
CH2
δ
CH2
γ
CH2
β
+H3N—CH—C
α
O
pK2 = 9.0
pK1 = 2.2
O

2,6-Diaminohexanoic acid $C_6H_{14}N_2O_2$

Lysine has a positively charged ε-amino group (a primary amine).

The amino group is highly reactive and often participates in reactions at the active centers of enzymes. Proteins only have one α amino group, but numerous ε amino groups.

Lysine is often found buried with only the ε amino group exposed to solvent.

Methionine

α Amino methyl thio butyric acid

SOURCE

Beans, beef, dairy products, eggs, fish, garlic, liver, onions, sardines, yoghurt, whey protein.

High quality proteins contain on average 26 mg/gm of protein.

FACTORS INCREASING DEMAND

Achlorhydria, alcohol, coeliac disease, digestive disorders, enteritis, exposure to vinyl chloride, pesticides, generalised hyper-amino aciduria, heavy metal toxicity, hypochlorite sensitivity, kidney failure, vitamin B_6 deficiency.

FUNCTIONS FACILITATED

Antioxidant, conjugation reactions, detoxifies endogenous epinephrine, norepinephrine and serotonin; free radical scavenger, involved in the synthesis of choline, acetylcholine, adrenaline, antibodies, carnitine, and creatine phosphate; involved in transmethylation reactions, lipotropic activity, precursor to cysteine, cystine & taurine; prevents oncogenic activity through methylating DNA, required for nucleic acid protein, collagen, polyamine & phosphatidyl choline synthesis.

DEFICIENCY MAY CAUSE OR BE ASSOCIATED WITH:

Atherosclerosis, choline deficiency, hepato carcinogenesis, hyper-cholesterolaemia, loss of appetite, poor immunity.

THERAPEUTIC USES

Ageing, AIDS dementia, alcoholism, allergies, atherosclerosis, athletes, bladder irritation, burns, cancer, chemical sensitivity, detoxification procedures, elevated lipids, fatigue, gall stones, heroin addiction, histadelic schizophrenics, kidney failure, liver disease, Parkinson's disease, pesticide exposure, irradiation therapy, reduce pancreatic cancer risk, surgery, trauma.

DAILY DOSAGE		
RDA	Infants	49 mg/kg body weight
	Child	22 mg/kg body weight
	Adult	13 mg/kg body weight
SR	Average intake 200-800 mg/day	

Note: reduce methionine levels in homocystinuria by supplementing with Vitamin B_6, B_{12} and folate to correct this imbalance.

TECHNICAL NOTES

SYNERGISTIC NUTRIENTS

Vitamin B_1, B_2, B_6, B_{12}, betaine, choline, cystine, folic acid, iron, magnesium, serine, taurine.

DISEASES LINKED TO AMINO ACID

Hypermethioninaemia.

DRUG/NUTRIENT INTERACTIONS

Paracetamol, Phenacetin.

ADVERSE EFFECTS AND TOXICITY

Increased red cell turnover and destruction, enlarged spleen and increase in weight of liver and kidney have been observed. Low protein diets with supplemented methionine result in a marked suppression of food intake and near cessation of growth. Supplementing with glycine, serine, retinol, vitamin B_6 and folic acid can reduce toxicity. Toxicity is due to the intermediate in the metabolism of methionine, called methanethiol.

Symptoms may include: severe nausea, vomiting, and hepatic dysfunction; de-creased serum folate and an increased white cell count.

PHYSICAL PROPERTIES

Non polar, hydrophobic essential amino acid, sulphur amino acid, insoluble in water, aliphatic.

STRUCTURE OF L-METHIONINE

2-amino-4-(methylsulfanyl)-butanoic acid $C_5H_{11}NO_2S$

Methionine is a sulfur-containing amino acid. The side chain is quite **hydrophobic** and methionine is usually found buried within proteins. It generally is not a participant in the covalent chemistry that occurs in the active centers of enzymes.

Methionine can react to form S-Adenosyl-L-Methionine (SAMe), which serves as a methyl donor in reactions.

Phenylalanine

2 – Amino – 3 – phenylpropanoic acid

SOURCE
Almonds, avocado, banana, brown rice, cottage cheese, eggs, fish, herrings, lentils, meat, nuts, pistachios, soybeans, whey protein.

Primary protein contains on average 73 mg/gm of tyrosine and phenylalanine.

FACTORS INCREASING DEMAND
Heart failure

FUNCTIONS FACILITATED
Appetite suppressant, constituent of enkephalins, precursor of tyrosine that leads to the synthesis of dopamine, noradrenaline, thyroxine and melanin; mood enhancer, helps memory and learning, stimulates the release of cholecystokinin and prolactin.

The **D-isomer** of phenylalanine inhibits enkephalinase (carboxy peptidase A).

DEFICIENCY MAY CAUSE OR BE ASSOCIATED WITH:
Behavioural changes, blood shot eyes, cataracts.

THERAPEUTIC USES
Agitation, alcohol withdrawal, appetite control, depression, kidney failure, memory loss, menstrual cramps, obesity, opiate withdrawal, Parkinson's disease, poor libido, vitalago.

D-isomers relieve chronic pain. D-phenylalanine is converted to phenyl ethylamine.

DAILY DOSAGE		
RDA	Infants	41 mg/kg body weight
	Child	22 mg/kg body weight
	Adult	16 mg/kg body weight
SR	Average intake 150-1200 mg/day	

EFFECTS OF OVERDOSAGE AND TOXICITY
Can cause anxiety and headaches.

Should be avoided in phenylketonuria and by women who are pregnant or lactating.

TECHNICAL NOTES

SYNERGISTIC NUTRIENTS
Vitamin B_3, B_6, C, copper, folic acid, manganese, iron, magnesium, zinc, chromium.

Phenylalanine excess may inhibit methionine transport across the blood brain barrier.

DISEASES LINKED TO AMINO ACID	
Phenylketonuria	Defect in the enzyme phenylalanine 4 mono-oxygenase.
Symptoms	Mental retardation, eczema type rash, lack of pigmentation in skin and hair, seizures, microcephaly.
Treatment	Low phenylalanine diet, tyrosine supplementation.

PHYSICAL PROPERTIES
Non polar, hydrophobic essential amino acid, aromatic amino acid, insoluble in water.

STRUCTURE OF L-PHENYLALANINE

2-Amino-3-phenyl-propanoic acid $C_9H_{11}NO_2$

Phenylalanine is a derivative of alanine with a phenyl substituent on the β carbon. Phenylalanine is quite **hydrophobic**.

Due to its **hydrophobicity**, phenylalanine is nearly always found buried within a protein. The π electrons of the phenyl ring can stack with other aromatic systems and often do within folded proteins, adding to the stability of the structure.

Proline

2 Pyrrolidine carboxylic acid

SOURCE

Most protein sources – beans, cheese, dairy products, egg, fish, pork, soy bean, whey protein, wheat germ.

Biosynthesis from glutamic acid.

FACTORS INCREASING DEMAND

Angina, ageing, inflammation, surgery, wound healing.

FUNCTIONS FACILITATED

A major component (hydroxy proline) of connective tissue proteins – collagen, elastin, tooth enamel; component of substance P, helps contain the loss of protein during aging, helps strengthen cardiac muscle, makes proteins heat stable, prevents lipoprotein (a) from binding to the vascular wall. Activates the pentose phosphate pathway, generates ATP for survival or ROS for programmed cell death.

Proline is a stress substrate in the microenvironment of inflammation and tumorigenesis. p53 activates proline oxidase (POX) proline dehydrogenase (PRODH).

Keeps muscle and joints flexible, promotes healthy skin.

THERAPEUTIC USES

Ageing, angina, atheroma, chronic back pain, heart failure, hypercholesterolaemia, hypermobility of joints, osteoarthritis, persistant soft tissue sprains, raised lipoprotein (a) levels, soft tissue injuries, tumor.

DAILY DOSAGE	
SR	500-3000 mg

TECHNICAL NOTES

SYNERGISTIC NUTRIENTS

Bioflavonoids, copper, iron, niacin, vitamin C, lysine, green tea extract, glycine.

PROLINE UTILISING ENZYMES

Proline oxidase
Proline dehydrogenase

INBORN ERRORS OF METABOLISM

Hyperprolinemia (type1) – due to a deficiency of proline dehydrogenase.

PHYSICAL PROPERTIES

Non-polar hydrophobic amino acid, heterocyclic amino acid, insoluble in water.

STRUCTURE OF L-PROLINE

Pyrrolidine-2-carboxylic acid   C$_5$H$_9$NO$_2$

Proline is the only cyclic amino acid. Formally, proline is not an amino acid, but an **imino acid.**

Proline is often found at the end of α helix or in turns or loops. Unlike other amino acids which exist almost exclusively in the trans-form in polypeptides, proline can exist in the cis-configuration in peptides. The cis and trans forms are nearly isoenergetic. The cis/trans isomerization can play an important role in the folding of proteins.

Serine

α Amino β hydroxypropionic acid

SOURCE

Most protein sources – beans, dairy products, egg, fish, legumes, pork, Ricotta cheese, wheat germ, whey protein.

FACTORS INCREASING DEMAND

Diabetes, corticosteroids, glucagon, hyperglycaemia.

FUNCTIONS FACILITATED

Constituents of phospholipids in the brain, involved in glycoprotein synthesis, phosphatidyl serine component of cell membranes, involved in the synthesis of pyrimidines, purine, creatine, porphyrin, glycine, sarcosine, choline and fatty acid sheaths around nerve fibres; increases the synthesis of immunoglobulins, neuro inhibitor, precursor of ethanolamine and glycine, glycogenesis, serine enhances the effects of opiates by increasing opiate binding.

Helps the synthesis of antibodies.

DEFICIENCY MAY BE ASSOCIATED WITH:

Serine deficiency mimics folic acid and B_{12} neurological symptoms, e.g. neuritis, neuropathy, behavioural disturbances.

THERAPEUTIC USES

Behavioural disturbances, chronic fatigue diabetes, fibromyalgia, haemodialysis, homocystinuria, memory support, multiple sclerosis, natural moisturiser, neuritis, neuropathy, pain relief, poor immunity, skin dryness (cosmetic agent), reading difficulties, spinal injury, uraemia.

DAILY DOSAGE	
SR	None given

Serine can exacerbate psychosis if vitamin B_6 is limiting.

TECHNICAL NOTES

SYNERGISTIC NUTRIENTS

Vitamin B_3, B_6, C, B_{12}, glycine, betaine, folic acid, magnesium, methionine, threonine, zinc.

DISEASES LINKED TO AMINO ACID
3 phosphoglycerate dehydrogenase deficiency is an inborn error of serine biosynthesis associated with seizures.

TREATMENT	
Glycine	200mg/kg/day
Serine	500mg/kg/day

PHYSICAL PROPERTIES

Neutral hydrophilic (polar), hydroxy amino acid, aliphatic, water soluble, electrically neutral.

STRUCTURE OF L-SERINE

$$\begin{array}{c} OH \\ \gamma \,| \\ CH_2 \\ \beta \,| \\ ^+H_3N - \underset{\alpha}{CH} - C \!\!=\!\! O \\ \end{array}$$

pK$_2$ = 9.2   O   pK$_1$ = 2.2

2-amino-3-hydroxypropanoic acid $C_3H_7NO_3$

Serine is a hydroxyl amino acid. It is **hydrophilic** due to the hydrogen bonding capacity of the hydroxyl group.

As a constituent of proteins, its side chain can undergo o-linked glycosylation.

It is commonly phosphorylated by kinases during cell signalling.

Taurine

2-aminoethane sulphuric acid

SOURCE
Present in animal protein (organ meats, brain offal, eggs, seafood), but not in vegetable protein.

FACTORS INCREASING DEMAND
Alcohol, cortisone, cytoprotective, epilepsy, essential hypertension, excessive intake of fructose, fluoride exposure, infants (formula fed), MSG intake, nursing mothers, oral contraceptives (estradiol), parquet exposure, protein malabsorption, soy milk fed infants, stress, vegetarianism, weight loss programs.

FUNCTIONS FACILITATED
Acts with glycine and gamma amino butyric acid as an inhibitory neurotransmitter, anti-hyperlipidemia, anti-hyperglycaemia, detoxifying reactions (conjugation of chemical toxins), facilitates the passage of calcium, potassium, sodium and magnesium ions in and out of cells; hyper-insulin effects, involved in bile synthesis, regulator of Na+K+ ATPase pump and calcium channels, stabilising the cell membrane electrically; reduces alcohol toxicity, regulates immunity by regulating hypochlorite synthesis in the neutrophil, stimulates growth hormone synthesis, stimulates prolactin and insulin release, spares potassium in heart disease, suppresses bronchial response to platelet activating factor (PAF), stabilises the excitability of membranes, osmo-regulation, acts as an antioxidant amino acid, modulates apoptosis of a variety of cancer cell lines, strengthens cardiac contractility.

DEFICIENCY MAY CAUSE OR BE ASSOCIATED WITH:
Cholestasis, cow's milk allergy, epilepsy, gall bladder disease, heart disease, high blood cholesterol, inflammation, lethargy, sleep disturbances, skeletal muscle damage.

THERAPEUTIC USES
Acute hepatitis, alcohol toxicity, alcohol withdrawal, anxiety states, asthma, brain seizures, cardiac arrhythmia, cardiomyopathy, chemically induced lung fibrosis, chemical sensitivity e.g. chlorine, aldehydes; ciguatera poisoning, congestive heart failure, cystic fibrosis, diabetes, Down's syndrome, endothelial dysfunction, epilepsy, fat malabsorption, Fanconi syndrome, formula fed babies, fatigue with VDV displays, gall bladder disease, heart failure, hepatitis, high blood pressure, high cholesterol, hyperthyroidism, jaundice, liver fibrosis, macular degeneration, mania, myotonia, neuropathy, naturopathy, platelet aggression, pregnancy, pre-term infants, poor fat digestion, reduces lead toxicity, retinal dysfunction, retinitis pigmentosa, retinopathy, sperm motility, spider bites, stress, sugar induced cataracts, valvular heart disease, vegans.

DAILY DOSAGE	
RDA	N/A
SR	250-3000 mg

TOXICITY
Non toxic.

May aggravate individuals with stomach ulcers, gastric upsets and loose motions.

TECHNICAL NOTES

SYNERGISTIC NUTRIENTS

Vitamin A, B_5, B_6, B_3, B_{12}, E, cysteine, folate, manganese, methionine, serine, tryptophan, vanadium, zinc.

PHYSICAL PROPERTIES

Sulphur amino acid.

DRUG/NUTRIENT INTERACTIONS

Alcohol, Bleomycin, cyclosporine, doxorubicin, herbal diuretics, morphine.

STRUCTURE OF TAURINE

2-Aminoethanesulfonic acid
$C_2H_7NO_3S$

2-Aminoethanesulfonic acid $C_2H_7NO_3S$

Taurine is a derivative of methionine & cysteine (L-methionine _ L-cysteine _ taurine). Taurine synthesis occurs in the liver and the brain. Taurine has also been found in extremely high concentrations in the brain, intestines and skeletal muscles.

Threonine

α Amino beta hydroxybutyric acid

SOURCE

Cheese, eggs, fish, lentils, meat, milk, pork, sea food. Low in most grains.

Primary protein contains 35 mg/gm of protein.

FACTORS INCREASING DEMAND

Corticosteroids, glucagon, intestinal malabsorption, renal failure, vegetarianism.

FUNCTIONS FACILITATED

Carrier for phosphate in phosphoproteins, copper transporter, essential precursor of glycine (neuro-inhibitor) and serine, immuno stimulant, involved in the synthesis of glycoproteins, lipotropic activity, plays a role in the formation of tooth enamel, collagen and elastin; maintenance of connective tissue integrity, precursor to the neurotransmitter glycine in the lower brain stem and retina.

Supports cardiovascular, liver, CNS and the immune system.

DEFICIENCY MAY CAUSE OR BE ASSOCIATED WITH:

Confusion, depression of feeding, digestive problems, emotional agitation, fatty liver, severe depression (epileptic drugs may lower plasma threonine levels).

THERAPEUTIC USES

Ageing, amyotrophic lateral sclerosis (ALS), detoxification reactions (via glycine), indigestion, intestinal ulcers, liver disease, fatty liver, motor-neuron disease, multiple sclerosis, NASH, renal failure, spasticity, spinal injury, spinal pain, trauma, vegetarians, wound healing.

DAILY DOSAGE		
RDA	**Infants** 68 mg/kg body weight	
	Child 28 mg/kg body weight	
	Adult 15-20 mg/kg body weight	
SR	Average intake 250-2500 mg/day	

Small neutral amino acids compete for its uptake in the brain.

TECHNICAL NOTES

SYNERGISTIC NUTRIENTS

Vitamin B_3, B_6, C, chromium, folic acid, glycine, magnesium, manganese, serine, zinc.

DISEASES LINKED TO AMINO ACID	
Hyperthreoninaemia	deficiency in the enzyme threonine dehydratase.

PHYSICAL PROPERTIES

Essential amino acid, neutral hydrophilic (polar), water soluble, aliphatic.

Glycogenic amino acid.

STRUCTURE OF L-THREONINE

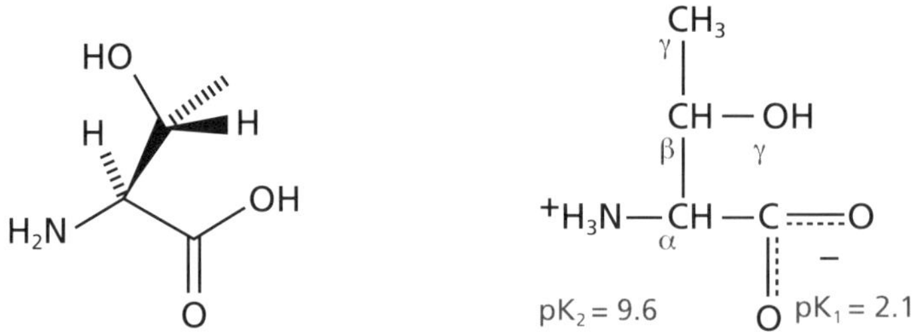

HO

H ...... H

H₂N

OH

O

CH_3

γ

$CH - OH$

β γ

$^+H_3N - CH - C \dashrightarrow O$

α

O

$pK_2 = 9.6$ $pK_1 = 2.1$

2-Amino-3-hydroxybutanoic acid $C_4H_9NO_3$

Threonine is hydroxyl-containing amino acid and is a **hydrophilic** molecule.

Both the α and β carbons of threonine are optically active.

The threonine side chain can be o-link glycosylated.

Tryptophan

SOURCE

Bananas, beef, beans, dairy products, cottage cheese, fish, legumes, lentils, oats, peanuts, pumpkin seeds, sesame seeds, soybeans, uncooked rice.

FUNCTIONS FACILITATED

Enhances nucleocytoplasmic translocation of mRNA, precursor of vitamin B_3, melatonin, & serotonin (5HT); stimulates liver protein synthesis, suppresses sweet craving and appetite, increases synthesis and secretion of GDNF and BDNF i.e. neurogenesis.

FACTORS INCREASING DEMAND

Aggression, insomnia, sweet craving, depression, excessive tyrosine intake, quinine intake.

DEFICIENCY MAY CAUSE OR BE ASSOCIATED WITH:

Anaemia, anxiety, cataracts, corneal vascularization, depression, decreased serotonin levels, decreased niacin levels, fatty liver, fibromyalgia, insomnia, neuroendocrine dysregulation, pancreatic atrophy, poor concentration, reduced plasma protein concentration.

THERAPEUTIC USES

Alcoholic aggression, AIDS, amphetamine abuse (drug addiction), anxiety, chronic pain relief, compulsive disorder, dental pain, depression, Down's syndrome, fibromyalgia, gut trauma, histopenic schizophrenia, hypertension, insomnia, impulsiveness, inflammatory bowel disease, mania, migraine, mild depression, obsessive compulsive behaviour, oral contraceptive use, Parkinson's disease, PMT, to reduce risk of sudden infant death syndrome, regulates appetite, stress, sugar craving, suicidal behaviour, uraemia, ulcerative colitis, violent behaviour, viral induced nutrient deficiency disease.

DAILY DOSAGE		
RDA	**Child** 12.5 mg/kg body weight	
	Adult 3 mg/kg body weight	
SR	Average intake 300-4000 mg/day	

Note: Tryptophan may be contraindicated in some individuals taking monoamine oxidase inhibitor drugs. It can aggravate aggressive behaviour. People with adrenal insufficiency or scleroderma should avoid taking tryptophan.

To increase transport of tryptophan across the blood brain barrier, it should be taken on an empty stomach with a sweet drink.

TECHNICAL NOTES

SYNERGISTIC NUTRIENTS

Vitamin B_2, B_3, B_6, C, chromium, folic acid, isoleucine, leucine, magnesium.

Phenylalanine, tyrosine, and valine compete with tryptophan uptake in the brain.

SIDE EFFECTS

Tryptophan contaminated during manufacture has been associated with eosinophilia myalgia syndrome.

DISEASES LINKED WITH AMINO ACID	
Carcinoid Syndrome	Tumours producing excessive amounts of serotonin with resultant tryptophan deficiency. Niacin may help.
Hartnup's disease	Due to a deficiency of tryptophan deoxygenase.
Symptoms	High excretion of tryptophan, pellagra type rash, mental retardation.
Treatment	High dosage niacin.

DRUG/NUTRIENT INTERACTIONS

Aminophylline, L-dopa, heparin, soprenoline, oral contraceptives, tegretol.

All these drugs increase free plasma tryptophan by increasing binding to albumin. Dilantin lowers blood tryptophan. Vitamin B_6 increases brain tryptophan levels.

Tryptophan supplements cause the reactivation of chlamedia from persistant to active metabolic forms. Giving antibiotics during the activation phase will increase the eradication of Chlamydia.

Quinine blocks uptake of tryptophan by brain cells.

Tryptophan supplementation causes the reactivation of Chlamydia from persistent into metabolic active forms. Giving antibiotics during the activation phase will increase the eradication of Chlamydia.

PHYSICAL PROPERTIES

Neutral hydrophilic essential amino acid, partially water soluble, heterocyclic amino acid.

Glycogenic and ketogenic amino acid.

5-Hydroxy Tryptophan

FUNCTIONS FACILITATED

Derivative of the amino acid tryptophan, immediate precursor of serotonin, reduces overall sensation of pain, suppresses appetite & promotes restful sleep.

THERAPEUTIC USES

Anxiety, cough, fibromyalgia, general muscle aches, impulsive tendencies, insomnia, migraine headaches, mild depression, panic attacks, restless sleep, unsocial behaviour.

DAILY DOSAGE	
SR	100-600mg/day

STRUCTURE OF L-TRYPTOPHAN

$pK_2 = 9.4$ $pK_1 = 2.4$

Amino-3-(1H-indol-3-yl)-propionic acid $C_{11}H_{12}N_2O_2$

Tryptophan is the largest of the amino acids. It is a derivative of alanine; having an indole substituent on the β carbon.

The indole nitrogen can hydrogen bond-donate and as a result, tryptophan, or at least the nitrogen, is often in contact with solvent in folded proteins.

Tyrosine

SOURCE

Almonds, avocado, banana, beans, dairy products, beef, cheese, chicken, egg, fish, pumpkin seeds, soy beans, wild game, whey protein.

FUNCTIONS FACILITATED

Component of enkephalin, improves concentration and working memmory, pigmentation of the skin; precursor of thyroid hormones, adreno-cortical hormones, dopamine, noradrenaline, adrenaline and melanin; increases alertness, regulates blood pressure, stimulates prolactin secretion.

FACTORS INCREASING DEMAND

Adrenal stress, brain fatigue.

DEFICIENCY MAY CAUSE
OR BE ASSOCIATED WITH:

Low blood pressure, low body temperature, restless legs, stress, exhaustion.

THERAPEUTIC USES

Adrenal exhaustion, alcohol withdrawal, Alzheimer's disease, appetite control, brain fatigue, chronic fatigue, codeine or amphetamine addiction, cold stress, depression, Down syndrome, drug withdrawal, environmental stress, haemorrhage, hypertension and hypotension i.e. it normalises blood pressure, hypothyroidism, improves sympathetic tone, mental endurance, mental exhaustion, Parkinson's disease, premenstrual tension, poor libido, phenylketonuria, restless legs, shock, smoking addiction, weight loss, ventricular fibrillation.

DAILY DOSAGE	
RDA	1120 mg
SR	400-6000 mg

(Care must be taken if given in conjunction with monoamine oxidase inhibitors).

Do not give to patients with melanoma or glioblastoma.

EFFECTS OF OVERDOSAGE AND TOXICITY
Dosage greater than 3% of the diet may result in corneal lesions, eye problems, palm and sole erosion and skin lesions. Not compatible with monoamine oxidase inhibitors. Toxicity reduced by supplementing with lysine, methionine, threonine or a high protein diet.

TECHNICAL NOTES

SYNERGISTIC NUTRIENTS

Vitamin B_3, B_6, C, biopterin, chromium, copper, folic acid, iodine, phenylalanine, selenium, zinc, 5HT.

Brain uptake is decreased by isoleucine, leucine, phenylalanine, tryptophan and valine.

GENETIC DISEASES LINKED TO AMINO ACIDS	
Pheochromocytoma	excessive tyrosine decarboxylase activity converts tyrosine to catecholamines.
Tyrosinemia (Type 1)	defect in hydrophenyl pyruvate oxidase.
Tyrosinemia (Type 2)	defect in tyrosine amino transferase.

Both result in raised blood and urine tyrosine levels.

PHYSICAL PROPERTIES

Aromatic amino acid, essential amino acid, neutral, hydrophilic polar, water-soluble, no electrical charge.

CONTRAINDICATIONS

Adrenal tumours, MAO inhibitor drugs, pheochromocytoma.

STRUCTURE OF L-TYROSINE

2-Amino-3-(4-hydroxy-phenyl)-propanoic acid $C_9H_{11}NO_3$

Tyrosine is an aromatic amino acid and is derived from phenylalanine by hydroxylation in the para position. While tyrosine is **hydrophobic**, it is significantly more soluble that is phenylalanine.

Valine

α Amino 150 – valeric acid

SOURCE

Almonds, beef, chicken, chick peas, cottage cheese, fish, lamb, lentils, lima beans, mushrooms, nuts, soy flour, whey protein.

First class protein contains 48 mg/gm of protein.

FACTORS INCREASING DEMAND

Cancer, muscle-wasting diseases.

FUNCTIONS FACILITATED

Calms emotions, enhances immune function of liver associated lymphocytes, improves muscle co-ordination, promotes mental vigour, prevents muscle loss at high altitudes.

Required for the synthesis of disposable amino acids.

Involved in globular protein structure with a preference for beta structures.

Competes with aromatic amino acids (tryptophan, tyrosine) for brain uptake; reduces brain tryptophan levels.

DEFICIENCY MAY CAUSE OR BE ASSOCIATED WITH:

Decrease synthesis of apolipoproteins, disaccharide enzyme deficiency, facial and vestibular nerve degeneration, fatty liver, hepatocarcinogenesis, myelin degeneration, negative nitrogen balance.

THERAPEUTIC USES

Alcoholism, anorexia nervosa, bad temper, body building, cancer, central fatigue during exercise, chronic renal failure, diabetes, dialysis, drug abuse, endurance exercise, hepatic coma, hepatitis, hepatoma, high altitude athletes, liver & gall bladder disease, muscle wasting, muscle weakness, poor muscle co-ordination, small bowel resection (acute phase only), sepsis, surgery.

DAILY DOSAGE		
RDA	Infants	92 mg/kg body weight
	Child	25 mg/kg body weight
	Adult	14 mg/kg body weight
SR	Average intake 500-5000 mg/day	

TECHNICAL NOTES

SYNERGISTIC NUTRIENTS

Vitamin B_1, B_3, B_6, magnesium, leucine, isoleucine.

NUTRIENT/NUTRIENT INTERACTIONS
Phenylalanine, tryptophan, tyrosine – compete with Leucine, isoleucine and valine, for transport into the brain.

DISEASES LINKED TO AMINO ACID	
Maple syrup disease	Deficiency in the enzyme keto – acid carboxylase.
Symptoms	Sweet smelling urine, vomiting, lethargy, seizures, resulting in death.
Treatment	Vitamin B_1, B_{12}, biotin supplementation and strict dietary control.

DISEASES LINKED TO AMINO ACID	
Hypervalinaemia	Subacute beta amino isobutyric aciduria.
Symptoms	Headache, irritability, delusions, hallucinations, crawling skin sensation.
Treatment	Avoidance of valine, reduced methionine and histidine, low protein diets, Vitamin B6 and magnesium supplementation.

PHYSICAL PROPERTIES

Non-polar, hydrophobic, essential amino acid, branch chain amino acid, not water soluble, aliphatic.

Glycogenic amino acid.

STRUCTURE OF L-VALINE

$pK_2 = 9.6$ $pK_1 = 2.3$

2-amino-3-methyl-butanoic acid
$C_5H_{11}NO_2$

Valine is an hydrophobic, branch chain amino acid. It is usually found in the interior of proteins.

Valine and **threonine** have roughly the same shape and volume.

CHAPTER 3

Minerals

All metals can cause disease through excess, deficiency, or imbalance. Malabsorption through diarrhoeal states can result in essential metal and trace element deficiencies. Toxic effects are dependent upon the amount of metal ingested, entry rate, tissue distribution, concentration achieved, and excretion rate. Mechanisms of toxicity include: inhibition of enzyme activity and protein synthesis, alterations in nucleic acid function, and changes in cell membrane permeability.

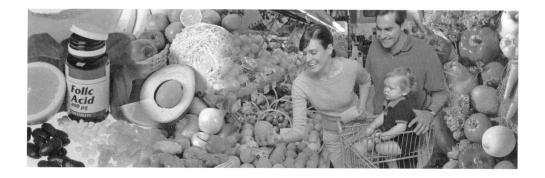

Boron (B)

SOURCE

Almonds, apples, dates, drinking water, hazelnuts, legumes, peanut butter, pears, prunes, raisins, soy milk.

FACTORS INCREASING DEMAND

Vitamin D deficiency, fluoride toxicity, magnesium deficiency, methionine deficiency.

FUNCTIONS FACILITATED

Decreases peak insulin secretion from the pancreas, improves the production of antibodies, improves energy utilization, improves the development and maintenance of bone, involved in parathyroid hormone function, activates vitamin D through its action in the kidney.

DEFICIENCY MAY CAUSE OR BE ASSOCIATED WITH:

Arthritis, decreased manual dexterity, depressed growth, elevated alkaline phosphatase, increases calcium loss, inhibits bone development, lowered serum testosterone and 17 beta-estradiol, poor cognition, poor psychomotor function.

TECHNICAL NOTES

SYNERGISTIC NUTRIENTS

Vitamin B_2, D, magnesium.

THERAPEUTIC USES

Osteoarthritis, osteoporosis, arthritic pain, menstrual symptoms, poor memory.

DAILY DOSAGE	
RDA	**Adult** 2-3 mg/day
SR	2-10 mg/day

TOXICITY	
>100mg/kg food intake:	Dermatitis, diarrhoea, lethargy, nausea, riboflavinuria and vomiting, chronic exposure, weight loss, decreased sexual activity, headache, hypothermia, skin loss, restlessness, kidney damage.
Acute Lethal Toxic Dose	18-20 g

Death due to circulatory collapse and shock.

Calcium (Ca)

SOURCE

Almonds, broccoli, bone meal, buckwheat, dairy products, egg yolk, green leafy vegetables, molasses, sardines, soybeans, turnips.

PROCESSING LOSSES

Water softeners remove calcium from water. Rhubarb, spinach, chard, grains & cereals, can decrease the absorption of calcium.

FACTORS INCREASING DEMAND

Alcohol, bed rest, bone fractures, caffeine, chronic vitamin C deficiency, diarrhoea, diabetes, diuretic use, depression, ageing, excess intake of fat, high blood pressure, high phosphate intake, high protein and sugar diets, high sodium intake, hypoglycaemia, hypothyroidism, intestinal malabsorption, inactive parathyroid activity, kidney disease or chronic renal failure, lack of exercise, lactation, magnesium deficiency, pregnancy.

Achlorhydria, age and excessive phosphate intake affect absorption.

Eating foods that bind calcium: Rhubarb, spinach, chard, cereal grains rich in phytic acid.

High or excessive intakes of zinc, magnesium, iron, sodium and manganese.

FUNCTIONS FACILITATED

Activates insulin, calcitonin and thyroid hormone release; blood clotting, bone and tooth formation, cell membrane permeability, cell signalling bio mineralization, decreases blood levels of parathyroid hypertensive factor (PHF), decreases cellular proliferation, maintenance of electrolyte, blood acid and alkali balance; muscle contraction, nerve transmission, regulation of cell division and hormone secretion, regulates heart beat, suppresses parathyroid and vitamin D action on vascular smooth muscle.

DEFICIENCY MAY CAUSE OR BE ASSOCIATED WITH:

Agitation, anxiety, ADHD, back pain, brittle finger nails, cognitive impairment, convulsions, delusions, depression, eczema, heart palpitation, hyperactivity, hyperirritability, hypertension (salt sensitive type), hypoparathyroidism, increased levels of parathyroid hypertensive factor (PHF), insomnia, irritability, laryngospasm, lead exposure, limb numbness, lower back pain, menstrual cramps, muscular cramps, osteoporosis, osteomalacia, paraesthesia, parathyroid hyperplasia, periodontal disease, PMS depression, rickets, sciatica, spinal curvature, stunted growth, tetany, tooth decay and loss.

THERAPEUTIC USES

Anxiety, arthritis, backache, bone pain, colon cancer, cramps, high parathyroid hypertensive factor (PHF) levels, hypertension, lead toxicity or exposure, menopausal symptoms, menstrual cramps, night muscle cramps, osteoporosis, osteomalacia, psychiatric patients, rheumatoid arthritis.

DAILY DOSAGE	
RDA	800-1400 mg
SR	1000-2500 mg
Deficiency limits	<200 mg

Approximately 45% of the population is at risk of being calcium deficient.

Citrate or malate forms of calcium have good absorption profiles.

EFFECTS OF OVERDOSAGE AND TOXICITY

Anorexia, anxiety, asthma, ataxia, constipation, depression, exhaustion, fatigue, flatulence, headaches, increased viral infections, memory impairment, muscle weakness, panic attacks.

These symptoms occur mainly in individuals that have a slow metabolism. Approximately 80% of the population are slow metabolisers.

Individuals who have high tissue accumulations of calcium are at risk of viral infections. Epstein Bar Virus is activated by calcium. This may lead to an increased incidence of chronic fatigue.

May increase the requirement formagnesium.

Calcium to phosphorous ratio – >2:1 results in reduced bone strength and interferes with vitamin K synthesis and/or absorption.

>2 gm – may cause primary hyperparathyroidism.

A high calcium to Magnesium ratio results in an increase in muscle aches and pains as does increased urinary frequency or urgency.

Hypercalcaemia as observed in cancer patients is associated with the following: excessive thirst, mouth dryness, dysphagia, dyspepsia, fatigue, gall stones, kidney stones, muscle aches, memory loss, tendonitis, depression, fatigue, restless legs, constipation or joint swelling.

Hyperglycaemia symptoms are seen in such diseases as Paget's disease, Addison's disease, individuals that are immobilised for long periods, hyperparathyroidism, malignancy.

Low thyroid and adrenal insufficiencies are commonly found in individuals with elevated tissue calcium.

TECHNICAL NOTES

SYNERGISTIC NUTRIENTS
Vitamin A, C, E, D, K, arginine, boron, carnosine, chromium, copper, lysine, magnesium, phosphrus, selenium.

HEAVY METAL ANTAGONISTS
Lead, cadmium

SITE OF INTESTINAL ABSORPTION
Duodenum, upper jejunum.

DRUG/NUTRIENT INTERACTIONS

Calcium decreases the absorption of these drugs:
   Tetracycline antibiotics – tetracycline, demeclocycline, doxycycline, minocycline, oxytetracycline
   Fluoroquinolone Antibiotics – ciprofloxacin, norfloxacin, ofloxacin, levofloxacin, moxifloxacin, gatifloxacin, lomefloxacin, sparfloxacin, trovafloxacin, alatrofloxacin
   Levothyroxine

Drugs that deplete body calcium levels:
   Aminoglycosides – streptomycin, kenamycin, gentamicin, neomycin, paromomycin, tobramycin

Amphotericin B, cholestyramine, cholchicine, digoxin, cimetidine, isoniazid, caffeine, digoxin, doxycycline, diphosphates, diuretics, fatty acids, fibre, oxalates, fluoride, methotrexate, mineral oil, neomycin, phenobarbitol, excess protein
   Anticonvulsants – phenytoin, carbamazepine, primidone, gabapentin, valproic acid, felbamate, lamotrigine, mephenytoin, fosphenytoin, clonazepam, ethosuximide, diazepam, clorazepate dipotassium, levatiracetam, tiagabine, topiramate, methsuximide, phensuximide, trimethadione, magnesium sulfate, acetazolamide, oxcarbazepine, zonisamide, ethotoin.

Salicylates – aspirin, choline salicylate, sodium salicylate, magnesium salicylate, salsalate, diflunisal, sodium thiosalicylate.

Corticosteroid medications – prednisone, hydrocortisone, methylprednisolone, prednisolone, betamethasone, budesonide, triamcinolone, dexamethasone, cortisone, beclomethasone, flunisolide, fluticasone, fludrocortisone, mometasone.

Loop diuretics – furosemide, bumetanide, ethacrynic acid, torsemide.

Aluminum and magnesium containing antacids – aluminum hydroxide, aluminum carbonate, magnesium carbonate, magnesium hydroxide, magnesium oxide, magnesium trisilicate, aluminium, magnesium hydroxide sulfate.

TARGET TISSUES

All tissues.

ENZYME SYSTEMS INVOLVED

Activates bone, kidney kinases, endocrine adenyl cyclase, muscle troponin and ATP-ase, blood prothrombin, choline esterases, and pancreatic lipase.

DEFICIENCY SYMPTOMS AS RELATED TO METABOLIC FUNCTION	
Hyperirritability	Decreased neuronal transmitters.
Stunted growth	Lack of available calcium for bone growth.
Bone demineralisation	Parathyroid hormone action, to restore blood calcium.
Tetany, convulsions, laryngospasm	Increased neuronal permeability to sodium and potassium.

Chloride (Cl)

SOURCE
Kelp, celery, olives, salt, seawater, tomatoes.

FACTORS INCREASING DEMAND
Water overload, diarrhoea, vomiting, burns, wasting and trauma, Barter's syndrome, cystic fibrosis, diuretic use.

FUNCTIONS FACILITATED
Maintenance of extracellular fluid volume, acid base balance, osmotic pressure.

An anion that balances sodium, blood pH and kidney function.

Required for the production of stomach acid and transmission of nerve impulses.

Activates amylase.

DEFICIENCY MAY CAUSE OR BE ASSOCIATED WITH
Hypochlorhydria, contraction of extracellular fluid volume, metabolic alkalosis, potassium deficiency, poor digestion.

THERAPEUTIC USES
Addison's disease, athletes, Barter's syndrome, burns, cystic fibrosis, diarrhoea, diuretic use, excessive sweating, trauma, vomiting.

DAILY DOSAGE		
RDA	Adults	750 mg
	Infants	180 mg
	Child <1 yr	300 mg
	Child <9 yrs	600 mg

Chromium (Cr)

SOURCE

Asparagus, apples, beer, brewer's yeast, cheese, egg yolk, grape juice, liver, lobster, molasses, mushrooms, nuts, oysters, peanuts, pepper, potato, prunes, raisins, shrimp, wheat, yeast.

PROCESSING LOSSES

35-45% from refining flour.

FACTORS INCREASING DEMAND

Ageing, blood pressure, cardiovascular disease, excess intake of refined food and sugars, glucose infusions, high cholesterol, high phosphate diets, hyperglycaemia, lipid metabolism, mature onset diabetes, oestrogen therapy, physical trauma, pregnancy, strenuous exercise, stress.

FUNCTIONS FACILITATED

Component of glucose tolerance factor (GTF), corneal clarity, glucose metabolism, growth, ligand to cell membrane receptors, potentiates insulin function, reduces total serum cholesterol, triglycerides and apoprotein(b) and increases HDL cholesterol; regulation of blood sugar and cholesterol, decreases glycated haemoglobin.

DEFICIENCY MAY CAUSE OR BE ASSOCIATED WITH:

Adult onset diabetes, anxiety, aortic plaques, ataxia, atherosclerosis, decreased insulin binding, decreased insulin receptor number, elevated circulatory insulin, elevated serum cholesterol & triglycerides, fasting, fatigue, glycosuria, heart disease, hyperglycaemia, hypoglycaemia, hypertension, increased intra-ocular pressure, impaired glucose tolerance, infertility, low sperm count, neuropathy, peripheral neuropathy, sweet craving, weight loss.

THERAPEUTIC USES

Body building, coronary artery disease, diabetes, dry eye syndrome, elevated intake of glucose or refined carbohydrates, gestational diabetes, high blood cholesterol, hypertension, hyperlipidaemia, hypo/hyperglycaemia, insulin resistance infertility, mature onset diabetes, myopia, stress, sugar craving, trauma, vanadium toxicity.

DAILY DOSAGE		
RDA	**Adults** 50-200 µg/day	
	Infants 10-40 µg/day	
SR	100-300 µg/day	
Deficiency limits	<30 µg	

Approximately 56% of the population is at risk of being chromium deficient.

EFFECTS OF OVERDOSAGE AND TOXICITY
Cr (3+) is not toxic in acute situations. Chronic intake results in diarrhoea or vomiting, renal and hepatic damage.
Cr (6+) is very toxic – results in damage to the kidneys, central nervous system symptoms, gut ulceration, carcinogenic, liver impairment, convulsions, coma.

TECHNICAL NOTES

SYNERGISTIC NUTRIENTS

Vitamin B_3, B_5, B_6, glycine, insulin, magnesium, niacin, zinc.

HEAVY METAL ANTAGONISTS

Lead, vanadium.

DRUG/NUTRIENT INTERACTIONS

Increase excretion of chromium:

Corticosteroids – prednisone, hydrocortisone, methylprednisolone, prednisolone, betamethasone budesonide, triamcinolone, dexamethasone, cortisone, beclomethasone, flunisolide, fluticasone, fludrocortisone, mometasone.

SITE OF ABSORPTION

Efficiency of absorption 1-3% inorganic, 10-25% chelated.

Highest concentration – liver, spleen, kidney, bone, testicles, heart, lungs and brain.

SITE OF EXCRETION

Urinary tract.

DRUGS AFFECTING NUTRIENT

Calcium carbonate, corticosteroids, insulin, salicylates.

Phosphates – bind with chromium and reduce its absorption.

ENZYME SYSTEMS INVOLVED

Component of glucose tolerance factor, phosphoglucomutase.

DEFICIENCY SYMPTOMS AS RELATED TO METABOLIC ACTION

Atherosclerosis, increased blood cholesterol	loss of insulin and chromium synergism.
Mild diabetes	poor insulin binding or action.
Impaired glucose tolerance, glycosuria	loss of synergism of Cr with zinc and insulin.
Corneal opacity	cornea concentrates chromium.

Copper (Cu)

SOURCE

Almonds, avocado, beans, broccoli, buckwheat, chocolate, crab, dried legumes, lamb, mushrooms, oysters, pecans, perch, pork, prunes, sunflower seeds, wholegrain cereals, water from copper pipes.

PROCESSING LOSSES

Variable

FACTORS INCREASING DEMAND

Ageing, achlorhydria, chronic bacterial infections, celiac disease, cystic fibrosis, excessive intake of alcohol, high intake of fructose, iron, sucrose, vitamin C and zinc; persistent infantile diarrhoea, low birth weight infants, malabsorption syndrome, pregnancy, potassium deficiency, short bowel syndrome, sprue.

FUNCTIONS FACILITATED

Angiogenesis promoter, antioxidant, cellular oxidation, catecholamine, myelin and melanin synthesis, clotting (factor 5), elastin and collagen synthesis, facilitates binding of opiates, increases the expression of tumour suppressor p53, maintains the integrity of the cardiovascular system, maintenance of skin, bone and nerve function; melanin and myelin synthesis, oxygen transport, participates in electron transfer in the mitochondria to produce energy, plays a role in synaptic vesicle to plasma membrane fusion, regulates iron metabolism, stimulates directional migration of endothelial cells, wound healing.

Co-factor in the activity of interleukin 1, basic fibroblast growth factor (bFGF), superoxide dismutase, cytochrome oxidase c, dopamine beta hydroxylase, ferroxidase, lysyl oxidase, phenylalanine hydroxylase, tyrosinase, monooxidase, tumour necrosing factor alpha (TNFa) and vascular endothelial growth factor and blood clotting factors V and VIII a component of ceruloplasmin (an acute phase protein).

DEFICIENCY MAY CAUSE OR BE ASSOCIATED WITH:

Alopecia, anaemia, aneurism, atherogenesis, bone disease, brain atrophy, cardiomyopathy, cardiovascular lesions (cardiac fibrosis, myocardial infarction with papillary muscle rupture) coronary thrombosis, coagulopathies, coronary thrombosis, decreased dopamine and noradrenaline levels in the brain, decreased longevity, decreased plasma enkephalin and CNS dopamine levels, decreased white cell count, demyelination of CNS neurons, depression, digestive disorders, emphysema, enhanced inflammation, enlarged heart, foetal resorption, fragile bones, general weakness, glucose intolerance, greying hair, hypertension, hyper-triglycemia, important for transferrin production, increase in serum amyloid A protein, iron accumulation in tissues, increase in peroxidation, glycation and nitration reactions, leucocyte production and bone formation; increased blood cholesterol, triglycerides and uric acid, increased susceptibility to candida and viral infections, infertility, iron accumulation in the joints, loss of myelin, Menkes disease, motor incoordination, neural tube defects, neutropenia, noise sensitivity, poor myelination, seizures, rickets-like bone changes, sparse, steely or kinky hair, spontaneous abortion, still births, tachycardia, weak blood vessels.

THERAPEUTIC USES

Alzheimer's disease, aneurism, back pain, baldness, bleeding gums, bacterial infections, cholesterolaemia, Down's syndrome, emphysema, excessive zinc intake, gout, haemorrhoids, High LDLs, hypertension, hyperglycaemia, iron resistant hypochromic, iron-resistant hypchromic microcytic anaemia, ischemic heart conditions, microcytic anaemia, iron storage disease, manic disorders, multiple sclerosis, poor iron assimilation, Parkinson's disease, osteoporosis (type1), pregnancy, premature infants, rheumatoid arthritis (due to iron precipitation in joints), sympathetic dominance, strokes, varicose veins, vitamin C excess.

Excessive copper exposure should be reduced in individuals suffering from glioblastoma, angiomas and metastatic spread of cancer. However it may help patients with Hodgkin's disease.

CONTRA INDICATIONS

Possibly cancer patients with metastasis, haemodialysis or chronic liver patients.

DAILY DOSAGE		
RDA	Adults	1-3 mg/day
	Infants	0.4-0.6 mg/day
SR	2-10 mg/day	

Approximately 25% of the population is at risk of being copper deficient.

EFFECTS OF OVERDOSAGE AND TOXICITY

Individuals metabolise copper at different rates, making copper toxicity an individual issue. The slower the metabolic rate, the higher the copper retention; regardless of copper intake. The higher the metabolic rate, the lower the copper retention.

Severe viral infections (mononucleosis, hepatitis) may cause copper retention, which may explain the fatigue, lethargy and depression associated with these infections.

EFFECTS OF OVERDOSAGE AND TOXICITY

Elevated copper levels also increase the risk of yeast and viral infections – Epstein Barr and /or cytomegleo virus, which contribute to chronic fatigue.

High tissue copper levels are associated with prolonged and heavy menstrual cycle. Zinc supplementation may reduce this heavy period.

Post partum depression is associated with elevated tissue levels of copper.

Zinc, vitamin A and C; are all antagonistic to copper and thus reduce copper toxicity.

>250 mg Acute	Coma, death, fevers, hypotension, liver and kidney failure, oliguria, tachycardia, uraemia.
>40 mg Chronic	Diarrhoea, dizziness, depression, dyslexia, epigastric pain, fatigue, general debility, green stools, heptomegaly, hypotonia, irritability, jaundice, joint and muscle pain, metallic taste, nausea, nervousness, partum psychosis, peripheral oedema, photophobia, PMT, premature ageing, wrinkling of skin, vomiting. High tissue copper levels can result in calcium accumulation around joints, causing aches and stiffness.
Wilson's Disease	Inability to maintain Copper status, causing accumulation in the brain and liver e.g. acute hepatitis which may become chronic, dystonia, dysarthria, dysphagia, drooling, open mouthiness, grossly inappropriate behaviour, psychosis, headaches, gold to greenish-gold Kayser-Fleischer rings or crescents in the eyes, amenorrhoea, miscarriage.

TECHNICAL NOTES

SYNERGISTIC NUTRIENTS

Vitamin B_2, B_6, B_{12}, D, amino acids, calcium, folate, iron, manganese, selenium, zinc.

Calcium and potassium increase copper absorption and retention.

Drugs that increase copper excertion

ACTH, alcohol, antacids (bicarbonate, Mylanta), corticosteroids, excess vitamin C, fructose, indocin, iron excess, Librium, lithium, penicillamine, phytate, oral contraceptive, tegretol, Thorazine, zinc excess.

Oestrogen increases tissue copper levels, while progesterone increases tissue zinc levels. An imbalance of these hormones can have a marked effect on tissue levels on these two trace elements. Excess oestrogen is associated with elevated tisuue levels of copper and low zinc levels. This may relate to PMS symptoms which echo copper toxicity symptoms of: frontal headaches, depression, fatigue constipation, emotional volatility, weight gain and food cravings.

At puberty, oestrogen levels rise, resulting in an increased tissue copper level, which may contribute to worsening of scoliosis at this time.

Tissue zinc/copper ratio may affect brain hemisphere dominance. High zinc levels in the left brain may predominate, resulting in better verbal, analytical and sequential thinking. On the other hand, increasing copper helps right brain functions, boosting creativity, yet it may also be associated with dyslexia; particularly if zinc levels are low.

Increase blood copper levels:
Estogens and estrogen like medications-estrogens, estradiol, estrone, estropipate, ethinyl estradiol, raloxifene.

Decrease body copper levels:
Colfibrate, fenofibrate, penicillamine, valproic acid, zidovine (AZT), ethambutol

NUTRIENT/NUTRIENT INTERACTIONS

Zinc, iron, Vitamin C lowers Cu absorption
Molybdenum increases copper excretion
Vitamin B6 deficency may decrease Cu absorption

SITES OF ABSORPTION

Small intestine, stomach.

Efficiency of absorption: 32-60%.

Minerals that favour copper absorption – calcium, cobalt, selenium, sodium and iron.

Concentrated in: kidneys, liver, brain, heart, bones, muscles and lungs (approximately 80-150 mg present in the body of which 10-20 mg is present in the liver).

SITE OF EXCRETION

Biliary tract.

Quercetin, zinc, molybdenum and vitamin C increase copper excretion.

HEAVY METAL ANTAGONISTS

Cadmium, mercury, lead.

ENZYME SYSTEMS INVOLVED

Carboxy-peptidase, cytochrome-c-oxidase, dopamine beta hydroxylase, histaminase, lysyl oxidase, most oxidase enzyme systems, neurocuprein, peptidyl-glycine alpha-amidating monooxygenase, superoxide dismutase, tyrosinase.

DEFICIENCY SYMPTOMS AS RELATED TO METABOLIC ACTION	
Anaemia	Loss of synergism with iron.
Bone and skin lesions	Decreased cross linking of collagen.
Demyelination	Decrease in phospholipid synthesis.
Defective pigmentation	Melanin synthesis blocked.

Iodine (I)

SOURCE

Asparagus, cod, dairy products, garlic, iodised salt, Irish moss, lima beans, mushrooms, oysters, sunflower seeds.

PROCESSING LOSSES

Refined foods are generally very low or devoid of iodine.

FACTORS INCREASING DEMAND

Diarrhoea, excessive carbohydrate intake, excessive weight gain, pregnancy, goitre, goitrogen rich foods – cabbage, turnips, Brussels sprouts, cassava.

FUNCTIONS FACILITATED

Cell division, endocrine modulator, mast cell immunoglobulin homeostasis, myelination and synaptogenesis, physical and mental development, synthesis of thyroid hormones.

DEFICIENCY MAY CAUSE OR BE ASSOCIATED WITH:

Accumulation of muco-protein, birth defects, breast hyperplasia, cognitive deficits, cretinism, decreased BMR, decreased plasma levels of T4 and T3, extracellular retention of salt and water, fatigue, goitre, growth retardation, heart disease, hypertrophy of thyroid gland, hypothyroidism, impaired protein synthesis, increased blood cholesterol, increased oestrogen-induced dysplasia, inhibition of trans-sulphuration pathway, infertility, insulin resistance, low IQ, myxoedema, poor motor coordination, ovarian cysts, polycystic ovarian syndrome (PCOS), syndrome X, tumours of the pituitary, weight gain.

THERAPEUTIC USES

Atherosclerosis, breast hyperplasia, cognitive deficits, cold hands and feet, goitre, hypothyroidism, infection, insulin resistance, obesity, oestrogen excess, ovarian cysts, polycystic ovarian syndrome, syndrome X, weight loss.

DAILY DOSAGE	
RDA	150 µg/day
SR	100-1000 µg/day
RDA by age:	
Infants	40-50 µg/day
1-3 yrs	70 µg/day
4-6 yrs	90 µg/day
7-10 yrs	130 µg/day
>11 yrs	150 µg/day
Pregnancy	175 µg/day
Lactation	200 µg/day
Deficiency limits	<50 µg

EFFECTS OF OVERDOSAGE AND TOXICITY	
>2000 µg Acute	Angioedema, gut irritation, hyper-sensitivity, hypothyroidism, serum sickness.
Chronic	Acneform skin lesions, brassy taste, burning sensation of mouth and throat, decreased thyroid activity, diarrhoea, gastric irritation, goitre, Grave's disease, head-cold symptoms, hyperthyroidism, increased salivation, increased sympathetic activity in the aged.

TECHNICAL NOTES

SYNERGISTIC NUTRIENTS

Vitamins B_3, B complex and C; NAD, copper, magnesium, tyrosine, selenium, zinc.

SITES OF ABSORPTION

All of gastrointestinal tract.

Arsenic, cobalt, iron and manganese influence iodine utilisation.

Efficiency of absorption 100%.

DRUGS/FOODS/NUTRIENTS INTERACTIONS

Goitrogen foods – cabbage, Brussels sprouts, legumes, tea, cassava.

Goitrogenine and Thiouracil – these interfere with iodine absorption. Sulfony-lureas, phenylbutazone, cobalt and lithium impair the uptake and release of iodine by the thyroid.

ENZYME SYSTEMS INVOLVED

Catalase, cystathionine beta synthase, myeloperoxidase, RNA polymerase, thyroid peroxidase.

DEFICIENCY SYMPTOMS AS RELATED TO METABOLIC ACTION

Decreased BMR – decreased synthesis of thyroxine.

Cholesterol, high lipid, salt and water retention – all due to decreased thyroxine synthesis and T3 production.

Iron (Fe)

SOURCE

Almonds, apricots, avocado, clams, liver, kidney, oysters, parsley, pine nuts, soybeans, sunflower and pumpkin seeds, poultry, red wine, wheat germ, yeast.

PROCESSING LOSSES

Variable

FACTORS INCREASING DEMAND

Achlorhydria, anaemia, copper deficiency, excess intake of calcium, haemorrhage, ingestion of excessive amounts of antacids, coffee and tea, pregnancy, senescence, excessive intake of dairy products, sugar and fat.

FUNCTIONS FACILITATED

Bone homeostasis, cofactor for monoamine oxidase, detoxification of peroxides, growth, haemoglobin synthesis, immune resistance, key element in respiration, skin and nail formation, oxygen transport, synthesis of neurotransmitters and DNA, activates telomerase, cofactor of monoamine oxidase.

Helps to convert phenylalanine to tyrosine. Low tyrosine levels are associated with lower thyroid function.

DEFICIENCY MAY CAUSE OR BE ASSOCIATED WITH:

Amylophagia (craving for laundry starch), anaemia (hypochromic microcytic), angular stomatitis, blue sclera, breathing difficulties, brittle nails, burning mouth syndrome, cold sensitivity, constipation, chronic dull headaches, deficit in cognitive behaviour, depressed growth, digestive disturbances, dizziness, dysphagia (difficulty in swallowing), fatigue, fearfulness, frequent need to clear throat, geophagia (clay eating), headaches, hyperactivity, hypothyroidism, koilonychia, left hemisphere neural deficits, loss of complex IV in the respiratory chain enzyme system, minimal brain dysfunction, mitochondrial DNA damage, mitochondrial stress, neurotransmitter disturbances, palpitations on exertion, pagophagia (ice eating) pica, poor appetite, poor immunity, sore inflamed tongue (stomatitis), spoon shaped distortion of the fingernails, weakness.

THERAPEUTIC USES

Anaemia, attention deficit disorder, brittle nails, cognitive deficits, colitis, fatigue, hypochlorhydria, infection, interrupted sleep patterns, learning deficits, menstrual problems, pregnancy, sore tongue.

Taurine reduced oxidative stress in iron overload.

DAILY DOSAGE	
RDA	10-20 mg/day
SR	15-50 mg/day
RDA by age:	
0-0.5 yrs	6 mg/day
0.5-10 yrs	10 mg/day
>10 yrs	12-15 mg/day
Lactation	30 mg/day

Approximately 25% of the population is at risk of being iron deficient.

EFFECTS OF OVERDOSAGE AND TOXICITY

>100 mg Acute	Biphasic effect, congestion of blood vessels, fatigue, headaches, pallor, pulse, rapid increase in respiration, in 6-8 hours – prostration coma, death.
Chronic	Arthritis, aggressive behaviour, anorexia, fatigue, gut damage, increased oxidative stress, cancer and heart disease, increased blood levels of serotonin and histamine, hostility, hyperactivity, headaches, liver damage, metabolic acidosis, Parkinson's disease, weight loss.

Note: 1:300 people have hemochromatosis – an iron storage disease.

Iron excess – reacts with citric acid, interfering with the Kreb's cycle and oxidative phosphorylation.

Activates xanthine oxidase and promotes the production of superoxide and uric acid.

Reacts with lactic acid and reduces its excretion, thus promoting cellular acidification.

Interferes with manganese superoxide dismutase.

Impairs the initiation of apoptosis.

Promotes or triggers mitosis and thus increases the risk of cancer.

Lowers brain serotonin levels over time, possibly inducing depression.

Promotes infection – allows Chlamydia pneumonii to thrive.

To reduce iron toxicity and its symptoms, supplement with: niacin, tryptophan, zinc, manganese, lipoic acid and quercetin.

TECHNICAL NOTES

SYNERGISTIC NUTRIENTS

Vitamins B_2, B_{12}, C, citrate, copper, folic acid, histidine, lysine, molybdenum and selenium. Copper is required for iron metabolism.

DRUG/NUTRIENT INTERACTIONS

Antacids (bicarbonate, Gaviscon, Mylanta), excess intake of zinc, manganese, aspirin, cholestyramine, colchicine, indomethacin, methyldopa, neomycin, tetracycline, penicillamine.

Decrease Fe absorption:

Bile acid sequestrants – cholestyramine, colestipol, colesevelam

H-2 receptor antagonists (decrease stomach acid) – cimetidine, famotidine, nizatidine, ranitidine.

Antibiotics – penicillamine, tetracyclines, neomycin, fluoroquinolone antibiotics (ciprofloxacin, norfloxacin, ofloxin, leofloxin, moxifloxin, gatifloxin, lomefloxacin, sparfloxan, trovafloxacin, alatrofloxacin, phosphorus.

NSAIDs and salicylate may increase the need for iron because of silent bleeding.

Salicylate – aspirin, choline salicylate, sodium salicylate, magnesium salicylate, salsalate, diflunisal, sodium thiosalicylate

NSAIDs – ibuprofen, naproxin, etodolac, flurbiprofen, indomethacin, ketorolac tromethamine, mefenamic acid, nabumetone, oxaprozin, sulindac, tolmentin, diclofenac, fenoprofen, ketoprofen, meclofenamate, meloxicam, piroxicam, celecoxib, rofecoxib, valdecoxib.

Stanozolol causes depletion of iron

HEAVY METAL ANTAGOISTS

Lead, nickel, mercury cadmium

SITES OF ABSORPTION

Duodenum, stomach, upper jejunum.

Efficiency of absorption 5-15%.

Ferrous form of iron is better absorbed than ferric.

Phytate in cereals, milk, cheese, polyphenols in tea, coffee, red and white wine, inorganic calcium, manganese, copper, cadmium and cobalt reduce iron absorption.

Stored in the bone marrow, blood, liver and spleen as ferritin and hemosiderin.

Total body stores of iron = 3.5-6 gm.

ENZYME SYSTEMS INVOLVED

Aldehyde oxidase, catalase (haeme), cytochrome C, cytochrome oxidase, mitochondrial α – glycerophosphate dehydrogenase, cytochrome P450, monoamine oxidase, NAD dehydrogenase, peroxidase, succinic dehydrogenase, tyrosine hydroxylase, xanthine oxidase.

DEFICIENCY SYMPTOMS AS RELATED TO METABOLIC ACTION	
Behavioural problems	Decrease in dopamine receptors in the caudate nucleus, impaired dopaminergic nerve pathway.
Listlessness, fatigue, anaemia	Decreased haemoglobin synthesis and lack of iron synergism with B complex.
Neurological symptoms	Decrease in brain aldehyde oxidase activity and increased levels of serotonin and serotonin metabolites.
Poor immunity	Decreased synthesis of anti-bodies.
Sore tongue, angular stomatitas	Lack of synergism with B_2.

Magnesium (Mg)

SOURCE

Almonds, barley, brewer's yeast, cashews, cocoa, cod, lima beans, figs, mineral water, molasses, parsnips, soy beans, wholegrain cereals, kelp, eggs, seeds.

PROCESSING LOSSES

Milling of wheat – 90%.

FACTORS INCREASING DEMAND

Achlorhydria, alcoholic cirrhosis, athletes, arthritis, bowel resection, chronic alcoholism, chronic fatigue, coffee excess, diabetic acidosis, diarrhoea, diabetes (type-2), eclampsia, emotional stress, epileptics, heart failure, high cereal intake or excessive phytate intake, high fat and sugar intake, hyperparathyroidism, kidney stones, lactation, liver cirrhosis, malignant osteolytic bone disease, microvascular surgery, muscular dysfunction, noisy environments, pancreatitis, pregnancy, pregnancy induced hypertension, prolonged diarrhoea, radiation, renal dysfunction, soft tissue calcification, sprue.

FUNCTIONS FACILITATED

Acetylation of CoA, aggregation of ribosomes, binding of RNA to ribosomes, cofactor in the synthesis of cAMP and ATP, cofactor and stimulator of many enzymes in energy producing pathways, cofactor in nucleotide excision repair, base excision repair and miss-match repair (DNA repairase), homeostasis of calcium, hydrolysis of phosphate and pyrophosphate, improves immune competence by removal of transformed cells associated with lympholeukaemia and bone tumours, improves insulin sensitivity and arterial compliance, inhibition of platelet aggregation, initiation of fatty acid oxidation, lecithin production, maintenance of heart muscle, muscle contraction, neuromuscular transmission and bone structure, regulation of body temperature, regulates intracellular calcium, sodium, potassium ions and pH; vasodilation of blood vessels, DNA replication.

DEFICIENCY MAY CAUSE OR BE ASSOCIATED WITH:

Addiction, agitation, anaemia (haemolytic), anxiety, arteriosclerosis, ataxia, behavioural disturbances, cold hands and feet, calcification of arteries, chronic fatigue, confusion, convulsive seizures, coronary artery spasm, decreased membrane integrity, depression, disturbance of heart rhythm, enhanced free radical damage, enhanced inflammation, hypothermia, hypertension, increased oxidative stress, insomnia, IQ loss, irritability, irregular heart beat, kidney stones, myocardial infarction, neurotic behaviour, palpitations, poor appetite, premenstrual tension, pronounced startle response, osteoporosis, radiation therapy, stomach acidity, talkativeness, tremors, vertigo.

Deficiency associated with decreased synthesis of PGE1, elevated PGE_2, substance P and CRP levels, which gives rise to neurogenic inflammation.

When magnesium deficiency exists, excessive amounts of calcium can build up in soft tissues, tendons, and ligaments; resulting in stiffness, arthritic and joint pain, vascular spasm or calcium deposits in vascular walls, kidney and gall stones.

THERAPEUTIC USES

Alcoholism, adrenal hyperactivity, allergic rhinitis, angina, anxiety, apathy, arteriosclerosis, asthma, asthenia, athletes, atheroma, aversions, bursitis, cadmium induced hypertension, calcium spurs, cardiac conditions, chronic fatigue syndrome, cocaine, constipation, convulsions, alcohol, and tobacco abuse; depression, confusion, diabetes, discontent, eclampsia, excessive, perspiration, fluid retention, gall stones, headaches, heart disease, hypertension, hyperparathyroidism, hyperactivity, hyper-excitability, hyper-sensitivity to calcium, hypothermia, insulin resistance, insomnia, insecurity, irregular heart beat, irritability, kidney stones, muscle cramps on exertion, muscular tremor, noise sensitivity, non alcoholic steatohepatitis (NASH), osteoporosis, osteoarthritis, palpitations, parathyroid dysfunction, premenstrual tension, pronounced startle response, protects from noise induced hearing loss, radiation therapy, renal dysfunction, restless legs syndrome, short term memory loss, stomach acidity or aches, stress, stroke prevention, suicidal ideation, sulkiness, tetany, tonic or facial seizures, traumatic brain injury, urinary frequency, vertigo.

DAILY DOSAGE

RDA	350 mg/day
SR	300-800 mg/day
RDA by age:	
0-0.5 yrs	40 mg/day
0.5-1 yr	60 mg/day
1-3 yrs	80 mg/day
4-6 yrs	120 mg/day
7-10 yrs	170 mg/day
11-14 yrs	280 mg/day
>14 yrs	300-450 mg/day
Lactation	355 mg/day
Deficiency limits	<85 mg
Deficiency markers	Plasma Mg <0.7mmol/l RBC Mg <2.3 mmol/l or < 6umol/g Hb

Approximately 49% of the population is at risk of being magnesium deficient.

EFFECTS OF OVERDOSAGE AND TOXICITY

>15 gm Acute	Acute Cardiovascular centres, malaise, nausea, paralysis of CNS, purgative, respiratory, sedation.
Chronic	Confusion, dry mouth, flushing, hypotension, muscle weakness, sedation, thirst.

TECHNICAL NOTES

SYNERGISTIC NUTRIENTS

Vitamins B_1, B_6, C, D, glucose polymer, potassium, boron, calcium.

HEAVY METAL ANTAGONISTS

Lead, Cadmium

SITES OF ABSORPTION

Duodenum, ileum.

Efficiency 30-40%.

Concentrated storage site – bone, muscle, liver, pancreas and non-muscle soft tissue.

70% of the tissue magnesium is stored in bones and teeth.

DRUG/NUTRIENT INTERACTIONS

Decrease magnesium absorption:
  Penacillamine, tetracycline- demeclocycline, doxycycline, minocycline, oxytetracycline

Increase excretion:
  Aminoglycosides – streptomycin, kenamycin, gentamicin, neomycin, paromomycin, tobramycin
  Amphoteracin B, Cholestyramine, Foscarnet, Digoxin, Cisplatin
  Loop Diuretics – furosemide, bumetanide, ethacrynic acid, torsemide

Thiazide Diuretics – hydrochloro-thiazide, chlorothiazide, indapamide, metolazone, chlorthalidone, hydroflume-thiazide, polythiazide, trichlormethiazide, benzthiazide, methyclothiazide, bendroflumethiazide

Decrease blood magnesium levels:
Corticosteroids – prednisone, hydrocortisone, methylprednisolone, prednisolone, betamethasone, triamcinolone, dexamethsone, cortisone, cortisone, beclomethasone, flunisolide.
Oral contraceptives – norethinodrone, ethynodiol diacetate, ethinyl estradiol, drospirenone, desogestrel, leveonorgestrel

Decrease body magnesium levels:
Hormone replacement therapy – estrodiol, estrone, estropipate, ethinyl estradiol, progesterone, medroxyprogesterone, hydroxyprogesterone, norethindrone, conjugated and esterified estrogens.
Pentamidine, Alcohol, Aldosterone, Ammonium Chloride, Beta Adrenergic Agonists, Caffeine, Cardiac Glycosides, Cyclophosphamide, Gentamycin, Laxatives, Phenobarbital, Riboflavin, Thyroxine.

NUTRIENT/NUTRIENT INTERACTIONS

Calcium and phosphate can reduce Magnesium absorption

Iron and manganese reduce magnesium absorption.

An excess of **vitamin B_1, C, E, and B_6,** has a stimulating effect on metabolism and increases magnesium requirement.

ENZYME SYSTEMS INVOLVED

Cofactor to: carboxylases, delta-6-desaturase, enolases, myokinase, glucokinase, isocitric dehydrogenase, peptidases, phosphokinases, phosphatases, pyruvate oxidase, thiokinase.

DEFICIENCY SYMPTOMS AS RELATED TO METABOLIC ACTION

Convulsions and hyperirritability	maintenance of nervous system and ionic balance.
Cramps	disturbed ionic balance in muscles.
Poor growth	Magnesium required for protein and DNA synthesis.

Manganese (Mn)

SOURCE

Almonds, avocado, beans, buck wheat, co-conuts, corn, kelp, liver, olives, organ meats, pecans, pineapple juice, sunflower seeds, walnuts, whole grains, turnips, carrots, broccoli, legumes.

PROCESSING LOSSES

Milling 80-90%.

FACTORS INCREASING DEMAND

Calcium supplements, Down's syndrome, congenital abnormalities, diabetes, epilepsy, pregnancy, vegetarianism

FUNCTIONS FACILITATED

Antioxidant properties (manganese superoxide dismutase), blood clotting homeostasis, bone and ligament formation, conjunctival pigmentation, enzyme activator and cofactor in lipid and carbohydrate metabolism, cofactor of hydrolases, kinases, carboxylases and transferases; enhances smooth muscle relaxation, intestinal enzyme function, mitochondrial integrity, mucopolysaccharides and cholesterol synthesis, otolith formation, glutamine synthesis, RNA synthesis, skeletal and cartilage formation, cofactor in the synthesis of thyroxine, prothrombin, dopamine and neurotransmitters; vestibular functions.

DEFICIENCY MAY CAUSE OR BE ASSOCIATED WITH:

Ataxia, adrenal insufficiency, atherosclerosis, birth defects, brittle bones, congenital malformations, convulsions, decreased catecholamine in the brain, decrease trigycerides and lipids, dermatitis, disc degeneration, disturbed carbohydrate metabolism, dizziness, epileptic seizures, glucose intolerance, hip joint dislocations, hypocholesterolaemia, hypothyroidism, impaired formation of otoliths in the inner ear, increased alkalinity or phosphate level, intermittent nausea, loss of hearing, nausea, non-trauma epilepsy, optic nerve abnormalities, osteoporosis, osteochondrosis, ovarian and testicular degeneration, pancreatic damage, Perthes disease, reduced fertility, sexual problems, skeletal and cartilage malformations, tendon and bone abnormalities, tinnitus, vomiting, weight loss.

THERAPEUTIC USES

Allergies, asthma, atherosclerosis, arthritis, cartilage damage, congenital ataxia, convulsions, diabetes, fatigue, hip dislocation in Down's syndrome, hypoglycaemia, knee osteoarthritis, low blood cholesterol, lupus, Osgood Schlaters disease, osteoporosis, Perthes disease, repetitive strain injury, schizophrenia, senile cataracts, sterility or infertility, tardive dyskinesia, tennis elbow, tinnitus.

DAILY DOSAGE	
RDA	2.5-7 mg/day
SR	2-20 mg/day
RDA by age:	
0-0.5 yrs	0.3-0.6 mg/day
0.5 – 1 yr	0.6-1.0 mg/day
1-3 yrs	1.0-1.5 mg/day
4-6 yrs	1.5-2.0 mg/day
7-10 yrs	2-3 mg/day
11-14 yrs	2-5 mg/day
>14 yrs	2-5 mg/day
Lactation	3-5 mg/day

Approximately 40% of the population is at risk of being manganese deficient.

Note: Patients with liver failure need to be careful with manganese supplementation as manganese is usually excreted via the biliary root. Manganese accumulates in the basal ganglia in these patients and thereby exacerbates hepatic encephalopathy or Parkinson's disease symptoms.

EFFECTS OF OVERDOSAGE AND TOXICITY	
>1000 mg	Anorexia, impotence, muscle fatigue and pain.
Chronic	Abnormal gait, anaemia, cirrhosis, compulsive actions, dementia, hypertension, hypertensive headaches, impotence, insomnia, mental confusion, muscle fatigue, nephritis, Parkinson's disease, paralysis, poor memory, schizophrenia, slurred speech, tardative dyskinesia, tremors, unaccountable laughter.

TECHNICAL NOTES

SYNERGISTIC NUTRIENTS

Vitamin B_1, C, K, biotin, choline, copper, iron, zinc, glucosamine.

HEAVY METAL ANTAGONISTS

Cadmium, lead, vanadium

SITES OF EXCRETION

Biliary tract

SITES OF ABSORPTION

Small intestine

Efficiency of absorption 3-10%

Iron competes with manganese absorption. Phytic acid (from cereal grains) and tannin from tea, binds manganese and makes it unavailable.

Concentrated in bone, liver, pancreas and pituitary gland.

TARGET ORGANS

Bones, liver, kidneys.

Total amount of manganese in body 20 mg.

DRUG/NUTRIENT INTERACTIONS
Corticosteroids, tetracyclines.
Fibre, phytates and poly-phenolic compounds may reduce manganese absorption.
L-Dopa – relieves manganese toxicity associated with Parkinson's symptoms.

NUTRIENT/NUTRIENT INTERACTIONS
Calcium and iron compete for manganese absorption.
Copper decrease manganese absorption.

ENZYME SYSTEMS INVOLVED

Arginase, cholinesterase, DNA polymerase, glutamine synthetase, glycosyl transferase, hydrolases, kinases, peptidases, pyruvate carboxylase, superoxide dismutase, transferases.

DEFICIENCY SYMPTOMS AS RELATED TO METABOLIC ACTION	
Ataxia	Myelin and mucopolysaccharide synthesis defects.
Hypoglycaemia	Defective maintenance of pancreas and insulin synthesis.
Impaired reproduction	Decreased cholesterol synthesis and hence sex hormone production defects.
Skeletal abnormalities, poor growth	Poor cartilage formation.

Molybdenum (Mo)

SOURCE

Beans, buckwheat, black eye peas, butter, kidney, lamb, legumes, lentils, lima beans, liver, navy beans, oats, oysters, organ meats, peas, pork, soy beans, sunflower seeds, sweet peas, wheat germ, yeast.

PROCESSING LOSSES

Major losses through the refining of flour.

FACTORS INCREASING DEMAND

High protein diets, excess copper and sulfate in the diet, metabisulphite sensitivity (symptoms of asthma), high tungsten intake.

FUNCTIONS FACILITATED

Anticarcinogenic; cofactor to a number of oxidase enzymes e.g. sulfite oxidase, xanthine oxidase, aldehyde oxidase; converts sulphites to sulphates, detoxifies carcinogenic xenobiotics, helps prevent tooth cavities, involved in fat, iron and copper metabolism; reduces angiogenesis, stabilization of the unoccupied glucocorticoid receptor, oxidation of aldehydes, purine and sulphites; purine metabolism.

DEFICIENCY MAY CAUSE OR BE ASSOCIATED WITH:

Asthma susceptibility, defect in sulphur amino acid metabolism, dental caries, elevated hypoxanthine and xanthinine excretion, gout, hypermethioninaemia, hyperuricaemia, increased susceptibility to sulphite toxicity, infertility, low uric acid concentration, mental and visual disturbances, oesophageal cancer, tachycardia (possible link to excess sulphite production).

THERAPEUTIC USES

Asthma (helps metabolise metabisulphite), cancer (breast, oesophageal, renal, stomach), candida albicans, infertility, exposure to pollutants, metabisulphite or sulphite sensitivity, nausea, perfume intolerance, sensitivity to fragrant & airborne odours, tooth decay, Wilson's disease (copper excess), yeast and fungal infections.

DAILY DOSAGE	
RDA	75-250 µg/day
SR	100-1000 µg/day
RDA by age:	
Infant	15-30 µg/day
Child <9 yrs	25-150 g/day
Child >9 yrs	75-250 µg/day
Adult	75-250 µg /day

Approximately 9% of the population is at risk of molybdenum deficiency.

Note: Patients with elevate uric acid or gout should restrict molybdenum intake to 75 µg/day.

EFFECTS OF OVERDOSAGE AND TOXICITY	
Adult	>2000 µg
Child 1-3yrs	>300 µg
Child 9-16yrs	>1200 µg
Acute	Severe diarrhoea.
Chronic	Anaemia (typical symptom of copper deficiency), copper deficiency syndromes, depression, elevated uric acid, gout.

TECHNICAL NOTES

SYNERGISTIC NUTRIENTS

Vitamins B_2, B_3, iron, sulfate.

Molybdenum and copper interact, share, or compete for common enzyme systems.

Sulphate competes with molybdenum for absorption from the gut.

SITE OF ABSORPTION

Intestine.

Efficiency of absorption 40-60%.

STORAGE AREA

Liver, kidney, adrenal gland, bone, teeth, skin.

Average body level of molybdenum 9 mg.

DRUG/NUTRIENT INTERACTIONS

Acetaminophen (molybdenum interferes with its metabolism)

ENZYME SYSTEMS INVOLVED

Aldehyde oxidase, sulphite oxidase, xanthine oxidase.

DEFICIENCY SYMPTOMS AS RELATED TO METABOLIC ACTION

Sulphite oxidase	converts sulphite to sulphate.
Xanthine oxidase/ dehydrogenase	catalyses the transformation of hypoxanthine to xanthine, and xanthine to uric acid.

Oxygen (O2)

SOURCE
Gaseous nutrient of air (21% of air).

FACTORS INCREASING DEMAND
Anaemia, asthma, breathing polluted air, cancer, chronic pulmonary disease, cigarette smoking, heart failure, high altitude, intermittent claudication, pleura effusion, poliomyelitis, emphysema, smoking.

FUNCTIONS FACILITATED
Essential for life, essential for mitochondrial function in the production of energy, enzyme systems involved – cytochrome oxidase, cytochrome P450 (approximately 350 different enzymes react with O_2), improves immunity.

THERAPEUTIC USES
Any condition that restricts the flow of oxygen to the tissues and cells. Reduces: metastasis, chronic lung disease, cardiac failure, emphysema, pleura effusion.

Tissue oxygen deficiency is associated with an increase in neoplasm or cancer.

DOSAGE
Maintenance of arterial partial pressure of oxygen is between 95-100 mm Hg.

TOXICITY EFFECTS
Irritated lungs, production of excess oxygen free radicals, oxidative stress and ageing.

TISSUE OXYGEN RANGE	
Skeletal muscle at rest	30%
Abdominal organs (at rest)	25%
Skeletal muscle during heavy work	86%
Brain (at rest)	20%

Phosphorus

(In its pentavalent phosphate form)

SOURCE

Almonds, beef, cashews, cheese, chicken, chickpeas, eggs, garlic, milk, nuts, offal, salmon, sardines, seed grains, sesame, soy beans, tuna.

PROCESSING LOSSES

No data.

FACTORS INCREASING DEMAND

Antacid abuse, calcium excess, coffee excess, diabetes, GI malabsorption, gluten sensitivity, growth, lactation, pregnancy, renal tubular dysfunction, premature births, total parenteral nutrition.

FUNCTIONS FACILITATED

Bone growth and mineralisation, buffering intracellular fluids, calcium homeostasis, component of DNA, RNA, phosphoproteins, phospholipids, energy metabolism & energy production (ATP); most B vitamins require phosphorus for activation, muscle contraction, phosphorylation reactions. Component of nucleic acid and phospholipids.

DEFICIENCY MAY CAUSE OR BE ASSOCIATED WITH:

Anorexia, anxiety, apprehensions, ataxia, bone pain, cardiac arrhythmias, chronic fatigue, familial phosphataemia, fatigue, irregular breathing, irritability, malaise, mitochondrial dysfunction, muscle weakness, numbness, nervous disorders, osteitis fibrosa cystica, osteomalacia, rickets, respiratory insufficiency, sensorimotor axonal neuropathy, skeletal demineralisation, susceptibility to infections, tingling paresthesia of tongue, fingers and toes; tinnitus, vertigo.

THERAPEUTIC USES

Alcoholism, diabetic keto-acidosis, fatigue, lactation, osteomalacia, pregnancy, rickets.

DAILY DOSAGE	
RDA	800 mg/day
SR	400-3000 mg/day
RDA by age:	
0-0.5 yrs	200 mg/day
0.5-1 yr	500 mg/day
1-10 yrs	800 mg/day
11-14 yrs	1200 mg/day
>25 yrs	800 mg/day
Pregnancy/ Lactation	1200 mg/day

Approximately 9% of the population is at risk of being phosphorous deficient.

Note: Phosphorus supplements are contraindicated in those with hyperphosphataemia and in those with severely impaired renal function (less than 30% of normal).

EFFECTS OF OVERDOSAGE AND TOXICITY	
> 4g/day Acute	Hyperphosphatemia, hypocalcaemia, hypomagnesaemia, laxative effect, tetany.
Chronic	Bone resorption, calcification of heart and kidney, osteoporosis, hypocalcaemia, secondary parathyroidism. Prevents the absorption of many minerals e.g. calcium, chromium, lung cancer.

TECHNICAL NOTES

SYNERGISTIC NUTRIENTS

Vitamin B complex, Vitamins D, B_3, calcium, magnesium, potassium.

DRUG/NUTRIENT INTERACTIONS

Anti-inflammatory steroids, Mylanta (aluminium hydroxide), excess iron or magnesium.

Decrease phosphorus absorption:
  Aluminium and magnesium containing antacids – aluminum hydroxide, aluminum carbonate, magnesium carbonate, magnesium hydroxide, magnesium oxide, magnesium trisilicate, aluminium, magnesium hydroxide sulphate.

Decreases body levels:
  Cholestyramine

Increases urinary excretion:
  Digoxin

NUTRIENT/NUTRIENT INTERACTIONS

Calcium decreases phosphorus absorption.

Iron and phosphorus bind together in the digestive tract and reduce the absorption of both.

SITE OF ABSORPTION

Duodenum, ileum, jejunum.

Efficiency of absorption 50-70%.

Concentrated in bone, teeth and muscle.

Adult body content of phosphorus is about 700 grams. It accounts for about 2%-4% of the dry weight of most cells.

Excretion is mainly through the kidneys.

ENZYME SYSTEMS INVOLVED

ATPases, cytochrome C reductase, dehydrogenases in oxidative phosphorylation, kinases, pyruvate decarboxylase, transferases.

DEFICIENCY SYMPTOMS AS RELATED TO METABOLIC ACTION

Osteomalacia	resorption of bone, decreased oxygen delivery and loss of ATP through deficiency of diphosphoglycerate, rickets.

Potassium (K)

SOURCE

All vegetables, apricots, avocado, banana, citrus fruit, dates, herring, milk, nuts (almonds, cashews, pecans), parsley, potato, raisins, sardines, sunflower seeds.

PROCESSING LOSSES

Variable – depending on the extent of leaching.

FACTORS INCREASING DEMAND

Adrenal stress, adrenal tumours, athletes, burns, cortisone therapy, dextrose and sodium chloride infusions, diabetes, diabetic keto-acidosis, diarrhoea, diuretics, excess intake of salt, coffee, tea, alcohol and sugar; hyperaldosteronism, hypertension (salt induced), laxative abuse, liver disease, malnutrition, renal disease.

FUNCTIONS FACILITATED

Blood pressure control, buffer constituent, homeostasis of eyes, secretion of FSH, ADH, and aldosterone; increases serum and urinary kallikreins, insulin synergism, intracellular acid-base balance, improves vascular smooth muscle function and structure, membrane transport, muscle contraction, nerve and heart function, modulates baroreceptor reflex sensitivity, natriuresis, osmotic pressure regulation, protein synthesis, hydration, regulates blood pressure, regulation of cell permeability and pH, inhibits platelet aggregation and the formation of arterial thrombi, maintenance of normal water balance, reduces vasoconstrictive sensitivity to nor adrenalin and angiotensin, prevents or reduces the incidence of cardiovascular or cerebrovascular accidents (stroke).

DEFICIENCY MAY CAUSE OR BE ASSOCIATED WITH:

Acidosis, acne, adrenal hypertrophy, bone fragility, bone and joint pain, cellular oedema, cognitive impairment, constipation, continuous thirst, death, decreased growth rate, depression, dry skin, fatigue, glucose intolerance, headaches, hypercholesterolaemia, hypo-reflexia, salt induced hypertension, insomnia, irregular heart beat, irritability, kidney damage, loss of weight, muscle weakness, paralysis, proteinuria, respiratory distress, rheumatoid arthritis, salt retention, sterility, stroke, tachycardia.

THERAPEUTIC USES

Adrenal hypertrophy, adrenal exhaustion, diabetes, alcoholism, as an antispasmodic, burns, diarrhoea, carbohydrate loading, cortisone use, cramps, heart disease, hypertension (salt induced), infant colic, liver disease, rheumatoid arthritis, weight loss, diuretic use, premenstrual tension, stroke prevention.

DAILY DOSAGE	
RDA	2-5 gm (50-125 m Eq/day)
SR	3-8 gm
Deficiency limits	<0.5-1.1 gm

Approximately 37% of the population is at risk of potassium deficiency.

EFFECTS OF OVERDOSAGE AND TOXICITY

>12 gm Acute	Cardiac arrhythmia, CNS paralysis, diarrhoea, fever, polydipsia, renal necrosis, tonoclonic convulsions.
Chronic	Cardiac and central nervous system depression, flaccid paralysis of extremities, mental confusion, tingling, weakness, cardiac arrest, kidney failure, dehydration, adrenal insufficiency, elevated plasma potassium levels.

TECHNICAL NOTES

SYNERGISTIC NUTRIENTS

Vitamins B_6, D, bicarbonate, calcium, insulin, magnesium, phosphate, sodium.

DRUG/NUTRIENT INTERACTIONS

Decrease blood potassium levels:
Albuterol, amphoteracin B, ritodrine, excessive intake of sodium bicarbonate, terbutaline.

Increase potassium excretion:
Aminoglycosides – streptomycin, kenamycin, gentamicin, neomycin, paromomycin, tobramycin
Corticosteroid medications – prednisone, hydrocortisone, methylprednisolone, prednisolone, betamethasone, budesonide, triamcinolone, dexamethasone, cortisone, beclomethasone, flunisolide, fluticasone, fludrocortisone, mometasone.
Salicylates – aspirin, choline salicylate, sodium salicylate, magnesium salicylate, salsalate, diflunisal, sodium thiosalicylate
Colchicine (by damaging gut mucosal surfaces); foscarnet, L-Dopa
Decrease body potassium levels:
Loop diuretics – furosemide, bumetanide, ethacrynic acid, torsemide
Calcium channel blockers – amlodipine, bepridil, diltiazem, felodipine, isradipine, nicardine, nefedipene, nimodine, verapamil

Thiazide diuretics – hydrochlorothiazide, chlorothiazide, indapamide, metolazone, chlorthalidone, hydroflumethiazide, polythiazide, trichlormethiazide, benzthiazide, methyclothiazide, bendroflumethiazide

Bisacodyl, Penicillins, Alcohol, Caffeine, Laxatives, Neomycin.

Increase potassium retention:
Angiotensin Converting Enzyme (ACE) inhibitors benazepril, captopril, enalapril, fosinopril, lisinopril, moexipril, perindopril, quinapril, ramipril, trandolapril) – ACE inhibitors will produce some potassium retention by inhibiting aldosterone production.

Potassium supplements should be given to those receiving ACE inhibitors only with close monitoring.

TARGET TISSUES

All tissues – mainly intracellularly.

Concentrated in muscle tissue and all cells of the body.

ENZYME SYSTEMS INVOLVED

Sodium/Potassium-ATPase, oxidative phosphorylation enzymes, some glycolytic enzymes.

DEFICIENCY SYMPTOMS AS RELATED TO METABOLIC ACTION

Bone fragility	loss of calcium synergism.
Cardiac problems	heart regulation lost.
Loss of weight	loss of synergism with protein, carbohydrate metabolism.
Muscle weakness	loss of nerve excitation.
Paralysis	high Na/K ratio paralyses nerves.
Sterility	loss of FSH function.

Selenium (Se)

SOURCE

Alfalfa, barley, broccoli, brazil nuts, butter, cashews, crab, celery, eggs, fish, garlic, human breast milk, kidney, liver, mackerel, oysters, peanuts, seleno-yeasts, tuna, wholegrain cereals, yeast, organ meats, onions, turnip.

PROCESSING LOSSES

Milling of grains 40-50%.

FACTORS INCREASING DEMAND

Ageing, alcoholism, cancer, cirrhosis, Crohn's disease, Coxsackievirus infections, cystic fibrosis, elevated LDL cholesterol, heavy metal contamination, hypothyroidism, Keshan's disease, premenstrual tension, pregnancy, smog exposure, smoking, total parenteral nutrition (TPN), vitamin C deficiency.

FUNCTIONS FACILITATED

Antioxidant activity, anti-tumorigenic effects, co-factor in the enzymes glutathione peroxidase, thioredoxin reductase, selenoprotein P, and iodothyronine-5-deiodinase; detoxification of chemicals, improves sperm motility & maturation, inhibitory effect on chemical carcinogenesis, facilitates the recycling of vitamins C and E, glutathione metabolism, inhibits lipid peroxidation, inhibits platelet aggregation, increases HDL:LDL ratio, maintenance of cellular membranes, maintains the activity of p53, modulates NFKb and AP-1 function, protects against chromosomal damage. regulates prostaglandin synthesis, spares vitamin E, stimulator of tyrosyl phosphorylation, synergises with sex hormones, stimulates DNA repair, thyroid hormone metabolism. Selenophosphate syntetase 2 involved in the synthesis of seleno P.

DEFICIENCY MAY CAUSE OR BE ASSOCIATED WITH:

Abnormal sperm motility, acanthocytosis, adeno-carcinoma of the bowel, cataracts, chondrodystrophy, confusion, deforming arthritis (Kashin-Beck disease), depressed CD4T lymphocytes, depressed glutathione peroxidase, depressed mood, growth impairment, haemolytic anemia, hostility, heart disease (cardiomyopathy), hypercholesterolaemia, hypothyroidism, infections, infertility, Keshan disease, liver damage, lung cancer, muscle degeneration, muscle pain and tenderness, neonatal jaundice, oxidative stress, pancreatic insufficiency, premature ageing, reduced lymphoproliferative response, sleep apnoea, sterility in males, senility and cognitive decline.

THERAPEUTIC USES

Adeno-carcinoma, ageing, AIDS, alcoholism, angina, arsenic poisoning, basal cell carcinoma, cadmium poisoning, cancer, cardiomyopathy, coxsackie viral infection, Crohn's disease, cystic fibrosis, depression, Down's syndrome, Friedreich's ataxia, heart disease, heavy metal toxicity, hepatitis-B-induced hepatoma, HIV infections, hostility, hypertension, hypothyroidism, inflammatory diseases, Keshan's disease (big joint disease), liver disease, reduces risk of miscarriage, multiple sclerosis, Parkinson's disease, poor immunity, prostate cancer, retinal capillary damage in diabetics, prevention of breast, colon, pancreatic, lung, bladder and prostate cancer; rheumatoid arthritis, skin cancer, sleep apnoea, TPN, thyroid disease.

DAILY DOSAGE	
RDA	50-200 µg/day
SR	200-800 µg/day
RDA by age:	
0-0.5 yrs	15 µg/day
0.5-1 yrs	20 µg/day
1-6 yrs	30 µg/day
7-10 yrs	40 µg/day
11-14 yrs	45 µg/day
15-18 yrs	30 µg/day
Adults	70 µg/day
Deficiency limits	<40 µg

Approximately 40% of the population is at risk of selenium deficiency.

EFFECTS OF OVERDOSAGE AND TOXICITY

>2 mg or plasma levels >100 µg/dl or >12.7 µmol/l

Arthritis, birth defects, brittle nails, dermatitis, dizziness, fatigue, garlic breath odour, gut disturbances, hair loss, Irritated eyes, irritability, hyper-reflexia, liver impairment, loss of fingernails and hair, metallic taste, mottled teeth, nauseas, peripheral neuropathy, vomiting, weakness, yellow skin.

TECHNICAL NOTES

SYNERGISTIC NUTRIENTS

Vitamin B_3, C, E, Co enzyme Q_{10}, cysteine, glutathione, methionine, zinc, iodine.

HEAVY METAL ANTAGONISTS

Silver, arsenic, cadmim, mercury, thallium.

SITE OF ABSORPTION

Duodenum, with efficiency of absorption being 44-70%.

Stored in liver, kidney and muscle.

SITE OF EXCRETION

Urinary tract.

DRUG/NUTRIENT INTERACTIONS

Reduce blood selenium levels:

Corticosteroids – prednisone, hydrocortisone, methylprednisolone, prednisolone, betamethasone, budesonide, triamcinolone, dexamethasone, cortisone, beclomethasone, flunisolide, fluticasone, fludrocortisone, mometasone

Oral contraceptives – norethindrone, ethynodiol diacetate, norgestrel, norgestimate, ethinyl estradiol, drospirenone, desogestrel, levonorgestrel

Decrease selenium levels in the body: Valproic acid, Anabolic steroids, chemotherapeutics, mercury diuretics

TARGET TISSUE

Kidney, liver, lung, ovaries, platelets, thyroid.

Plasma levels 8-25 µg/dl or 1-3.2 µmol/l.

ENZYME SYSTEMS INVOLVED

Aryl sulfatase, beta glucuronidase, iodothyronine-5-deiodinase, glutathione peroxidase, lactic dehydrogenase, oxalic transaminase, thioredoxin reductase.

DEFICIENCY SYMPTOMS AS RELATED TO METABOLIC ACTION	
Liver damage	Liver cell membrane damage due to oxidant stress.
Neonatal jaundice	Breakdown in red blood cell membranes.
Platelet problems	Cell membrane damage.

Silicon (Si)

SOURCE

Alpha alpha, barley, Bell's peppers, brown rice, horsetail plant, oats, root vegetables, whole grain cereals.

PROCESSING LOSSES

No data available. Losses are associated with over refining of food.

FACTORS INCREASING DEMAND

Ageing, arthritis, atherosclerosis, bone fractures, growth, hypertension, low oestrogen status, musculo-skeletal pain, osteoporosis, Paget's disease, weak nails and hair.

FUNCTIONS FACILITATED

Anti-arteriosclerotic, biological cross-linking agent, bone calcification, contributes to the architecture and resilience of connective tissue, decreases the infiltration of cholesterol into arterial walls, involved in the structural organisation of glycosaminoglycans and polyuronides, muscle contractibility, nerve transmission, plays a fundamental role in the cross-linking mechanism in collagen, elastin, and mucopolysaccharides; sodium pumps.

Involved in the development, growth and integrity of hair, skin, nails, and mucus membranes, arteries, bones, cartilage, and connective tissue.

DEFICIENCY MAY CAUSE OR BE ASSOCIATED WITH:

Aberrant metabolism of connective tissue and bone, brittle nails, defective endochondral bone growth, depressed collagen content in bone, long bone abnormalities.

THERAPEUTIC USES

Ageing, all arthritic conditions, aluminium toxicity, arteriosclerosis, atherosclerosis, bone fracture, bone mineralisation, brittle nails, cardiovascular disease, hypertension, musculo-skeletal disorders, osteoarthritis, osteoporosis, Paget's disease, pregnancy, tendon support, weak finger nails.

DAILY DOSAGE	
RDA	9-14mg
SR	20-50 mg

Note: High doses of silicon have been reported to form siliceous renal calculi.

TARGET TISSUE

Aorta, bone, eyes, skin, tendons, trachea.

ENZYME SYSTEMS INVOLVED

Bone prolylhydroxylase activity.

Sodium (Na)

SOURCE

Anchovies, bacon, bologna sausage, brains, celery, cheeses, clams, corn beef, liver, pickled olives, peas, pickles, table salt, tuna, salted butter, sardines, sauerkraut, processed meats, pasteurised cheese, potato chips, softened water.

FACTORS INCREASING DEMAND

Adrenal cortical insufficiency, chronic diarrhoea, coffee intake, dehydration, excess water intake, heavy sweating, lack of potassium, vomiting.

FUNCTIONS FACILITATED

Acid base balance, cell permeability, glucose absorption, elevated serum lipids, homeostasis of digestive and nervous system, maintenance of blood pressure, maintains water balance with potassium, muscle homeostasis, regulation of osmotic pressure.

DEFICIENCY MAY CAUSE OR BE ASSOCIATED WITH:

Abdominal cramps, anorexia, ataxia, diarrhoea, dizziness, fatigue, flatulence, hallucinations, headaches, heat exhaustion, hypertension or hypotension, muscle weakness, nausea, taste impairment, weight loss.

THERAPEUTIC USES

Adrenal cortical insufficiency, athletic endurance, cramps, dehydration, fever, vomiting, hot climate exposure.

DAILY DOSAGE	
RDA	0.75 - 3.5 gm
SR	3 - 9 gm
Maximum recommendation: Adult	2.4 - 3.0 g/day (Equivalent to 6 - 7.5 g of salt per day)
RDA by age:	
Infants	120 mg/day
Deficiency limits	<0.5 gm

Approximately 6% of the population is at risk of sodium deficiency.

Note: High salt intake increases platelet reactivity, stroke (independent of BP), left ventricular hypertrophy, cardiac heart failure and sudden death. It decreases renal plasma flow, increases glomeruli filtration and GFR, leading to an increase in intracellular capillary pressure, micro-albuminuria, proteinuria, glomeruli injury and renal insufficiency.

Sodium also reduces arterial compliance independent of BP.

EFFECTS OF OVERDOSAGE AND TOXICITY	
>18 gm Acute	Cognitive dysfunction, diarrhoea, excess salivation, excess water intake, exhaustion, fluid retention, hyperactivity, seizures, stiff gait, tremors.
Chronic	Anaemia, anorexia, fluid retention, hypertension, lipemia, polydipsia.

TECHNICAL NOTES

SYNERGISTIC NUTRIENTS

Vitamin B_6, vitamin D, bicarbonate, calcium, magnesium, phosphate, potassium.

DRUG/ NUTRIENT INTERACTIONS

Lower sodium body levels:

ACE inhibitors – benazepril, captopril, lisinopril, fosinpril, moexipril, ramipril, trandolapril, perindopril, erbumine

Salicylates and colchicine (by damaging gut mucosa absorptive surfaces and bleeding),

Loop diuretics – furosemide, bumetanide, ethacrynic acid, torsemide

Thiazide diuretics – hydrochlorothiazide, chlorothiazide, indapamide, metolazone, chlorthalidone, hydroflumethiazide, polythiazide, trichlormethiazide, benzthiazide, methyclothiazide, bendroflumethiazide

Bisacodyl, lithium, neomycin, cortisol, desoxycorticosterone, aldosterone, phenylbutazone

Estrogen and progesterone cause sodium and water retention.

TARGET ORGANS

Blood, lymph, nerves, muscle, saliva.

DEFICIENCY SYMPTOMS AS RELATED TO METABOLIC FUNCTION	
Anorexia, Nausea	Loss of gastric HCl and digestive juices.
Muscle weakness	Loss of neuromuscular irritability.

Vanadium (V)

SOURCE

Black pepper, chicken fat, dill seeds, corn, linseed, mushroom, parsley, rye, shellfish, seafood, soy beans, vanadyl sulfate supplements.

POSSIBLE FUNCTION

May play a role in iodine metabolism or thyroid function, regulation of some phosphoryl-transfer enzymes, vanadate (5+) ion is a potent inhibitor of Na+K+ATPase, is a component of several bromo and iodoperoxidases in lower forms of life, has a hypoglycaemic effect, can act as an insulin mimic, normalises blood sugar and reduces glycosylated haemoglobin in non-insulin dependent diabetes, increases the activity of phosphatidylinositol 3 kinase (PI3-kinase), increases amino acid incorporation in skeletal muscle.

DEFICIENCY MAY CAUSE OR BE ASSOCIATED WITH:

Deficiency states are unknown in humans. In goats and rats, it causes reduced growth, poor bone development, and impaired reproductive capacity.

THERAPEUTIC USES

Diabetes, elevated glycosylated haemoglobin, hyperglycaemia, insulin resistance, muscle building.

DAILY DOSAGE	
RDA	10 - 30 µg
SR	25 -100 µg/day

TOXICITY AND SIDE EFFECTS	
Safe oral ingestion	<2.5 mg/day: only 1% is absorbed from gut.

Inhaled vanadium is more toxic than when it is orally ingested.

Blood circulating levels 0.04 to 1 µmol/l (2-50 mg/ml) are associated with: depressive illness, gastroenteritis upsets, green tongue, manic depression, neurotic depression.

Vanadium dust exposure in the upper respiratory tract causes irritation, wheezing and nasal bleeding.

ANTAGONISTS

Vitamin C, choline, lithium, magnesium.

STORED

Kidney, spleen, liver, bone, testes and lung.

Total body stores 0.1-1 mg.

Zinc (Zn)

SOURCE

Beef, bilberry, brewers years, capsicum, egg yolks, ginger, herrings, liver, milk, lamb, oysters, sunflower and pumpkin seeds, sea food, whole grains, yeast.

PROCESSING LOSSES

Milling of flour: 80%, frozen peas: 25-50%.

FACTORS INCREASING DEMAND

Achlorhydria, acrodermatitis enteropathica, alcoholism, anorexia nervosa, bowel resection, burns, copper and lead toxicity, diabetes, elderly, exercise, high fibre diet containing phytate, hypertension, increased thyroid activity, poor appetite, pancreatic enzyme insufficiency, pancreatitis, pregnancy, prostate disease, schizophrenics, soy based milk feeds, sickle cell anemia, stress, tuberculosis, vegetarians, viral infections.

FUNCTIONS FACILITATED

Activates over 200 different enzymes in the body, activates tumour suppressor endostatin which inhibits angiogenesis, activates super oxide dismutase, anti-viral activity, brain development, DNA and RNA synthesis, helps the absorption of B vitamins, involved in over 80 different enzyme systems, cofactor in PGE1 synthesis, improves cellular and humoral immunity, maintains immunity function, increases the level of hydroxyl proline in wounds, inhibits 5-alpha reductase, maintenance of sensory functions, induces monocyte release of IL1, IL6, and TNF a; increases circulating leptin levels, improves carbon dioxide transport in the lungs, provides a structural role for regulatory functions, respiration, reduces lactic acid levels in overworked muscles, sexual development, supports insulin synthesis and action, synergism with growth hormone, wound healing (increases hydroxyproline in wounds).

DEFICIENCY MAY CAUSE OR BE ASSOCIATED WITH:

Acne, acrodermatitis enteropathica, alopecia, amnesia, anencephaly, anorexia nervosa, brittle nails, decreased leptin levels, decreased plasma testosterone, decrease immune response and increased susceptibility to viral infections,depletion of B-cell and T-cells, poor immunity, depression, dermatitis, DNA damage, growth failure, histological changes in cerebellum and hippocampus, hypercholesterolaemia, hypogonadism, impaired growth, impaired wound healing, impotence, increased developmental disorders, increased risk of abortion, learning disorders, loss of appetite, loss of taste and smell, low sperm counts (oligospermia), macular degeneration, manic depression,moodiness, neuropsychological impairment, neural tube defects, poor concentration, poor memory, poor vision, sleep problems,slow healing of wounds, sperm damage, sterility, stretch marks (white stretch marks indicate a relative deficiency, while red or purple stretch marks mean an absolute zinc deficiency), white spots on finger nails, viral infections.

THERAPEUTIC USES

AIDS, achlorhydria, acne, acrodermatitis enteropathica, acute diarrhoea, alcoholism, alopecia, anaemia, anorexia nervosa, apathy, arthritis, athletic training, autism, beta thalassaemia, burns, burning mouth syndrome, cadmium and copper toxicity, cancer, cirrhosis, coeliac disease, colds and flu, Crohn's disease, cystic fibrosis, dandruff, suppressed immunity, depression, diabetes, diarrhoea, Down's syndrome, epilepsy, fatty plaques, growth retardation, hearing loss, hyper-prolactaemia, hypertension, hypertriglyceridaemia, hypoglycaemia, hypospermia, hypothyroidism, infection, infertility, loss of smell and taste, night blindness, intermittent claudication, macular degeneration, manic depression, pancreatitis, pica, poor appetite, pregnancy, premature infants, poor libido, prostatic hyperplasia, prevention of prostatic cancer, psoriasis form of dermatitis, renal disease, rheumatoid arthritis, schizophrenia, sickle cell anemia, skin disorders, surgery, toxaemia of pregnancy, uraemia, viral infections, wound healing.

DAILY DOSAGE

RDA	15 mg or 0.2 mg/kg
SR	10-90 mg
RDA by age:	
Infants	5 mg
<10 yrs	10 mg
>10 yrs	15 mg
Lactation	19 mg

Approximately 47% of the population is at risk of zinc deficiency.

Doses >150 mg interfere with copper metabolism and cause hypocupremia, erythrocyte microcytosis and neutropenia.

Note: Zinc-histidine, zinc-methionine and zinc-cysteine complexes appear to be more efficiently absorbed than other zinc supplementary forms.

EFFECTS OF OVERDOSAGE AND TOXICITY

>1000 mg Acute	CNS depression, diarrhoea, dizziness, gastric distress, lassitude, leucopoenia, nausea, paralysis of extremities, slow tendon reflexes, tremors, vomiting.
Chronic	Abdominal pain, alcohol intolerance, anaemia, anorexia, cholesterol, dehydration, electrolyte imbalance, hypochromic, microcytic anaemia, impaired immune response, increased serum amylase and lipase, lethargy, nausea, poor growth, reduced HDL, symptoms of copper and iron deficiency, vomiting, suppressed immune function. Lowers tissue copper levels resulting in lipid abnormalities.

Nausea and emetic effect occurs: >150 mg Zn/day

TECHNICAL NOTES

SYNERGISTIC NUTRIENTS

Vitamin A, B_6, D, E, cysteine, glucose polymers, glutathione, insulin, magnesium, manganese.

DRUG/NUTRIENT INTERACTIONS

Decrease zinc absorption:

H-2 receptor antagonists – cimetidine, famotidine, nizatidine, ranitidine

Tetracycline – tetracycline, demeclocycline, doxycycline, minocycline, oxytetracycline

Increase zinc urinary excretion:

ACE inhibitors – benazepril, captopril, lisinopril, fosinpril, moexipril, ramipril, trandolapril, perindopril, erbumine

Corticosteroid medications – prednisone, hydrocortisone, methylprednisolone, prednisolone, betamethasone, budesonide, triamcinolone, dexamethasone, cortisone, beclomethasone, flunisolide, fluticasone, fludrocortisone, mometasone

DRUG/NUTRIENT INTERACTIONS

Loop diuretics – furosemide, bumetanide, ethacrynic acid, torsemide

Thiazide diuretics – hydrochlorothiazide, chlorothiazide, indapamide, metolazone, chlorthalidone, hydroflumethiazide, polythiazide, trichlormethiazide, benzthiazide, methyclothiazide, bendroflumethiazide

Penicillamine

Decrease zinc blood levels:

Oral contraceptives – norethindrone, ethynodiol diacetate, norgestrel, norgestimate, ethinyl estradiol, drospirenone, desogestrel, levonorgestrel

Valproic acid

Decrease body zinc levels:

Clofibrate, fenofibrate, ethambutol (particularly in heart, kidney, liver); zidovudine (AZT)

Alcohol, beta blockers, chlorthalidone, cholestyramine, cimetidine, EDTA, endopril, ethambutol, penicillin, pentobarbital, phytate (Inositol Hexaphosphate), polyphenols, progesterone, steroids.

NUTRIENT/NUTRIENT INTERACTIONS

Zinc and copper are capable of decreasing absorption of the other from the digestive tract.

HEAVY METALS ANTAGONISTS

Lead, cobalt, cadmium, nickel, mercury.

SITE OF EXCRETION

The major route of zinc excretion is via the gastrointestinal tract. Fecal zinc excretion is comprised of unabsorbed zinc and zinc derived from biliary, pancreatic, and gastrointestinal secretions and zinc from sloughing of mucosal cells.

SITES OF ABSORPTION

Duodenum, ileum, jejunum.

Efficiency of absorption 15-50%.

Approximate amount in the body 1.5-2.5 gm.

Absorption is inhibited by: excess sugar intake, insufficient stomach HCl and pancreatic enzymes, gut inflammation and allergy.

Excessive calcium intake impairs zinc absorption. Zinc competes with calcium and iron for absorption.

TARGET ORGAN

Brain, optic nerve, eye, semen, prostate gland, pancreas and adrenal gland.

90% of the zinc is stored in muscle and bone.

ENZYME SYSTEMS INVOLVED

Alcohol dehydrogenase and many other enzymes, alkaline phosphatase, catalase, DNA transcription factors, involved in the co-enzyme system, lactate dehydrogenase, NADH dehydrogenase, renal dipeptidase, RNA and DNA polymerase, super oxide dismutase.

DEFICIENCY SYMPTOMS AS RELATED TO METABOLIC ACTION

(Plasma <70 µg/dl)

Growth failure	DNA synthesis impaired.
Hypogonadism	Decrease in germinal epithelium.
Impaired wound healing	Mucopolysaccharide synthesis is decreased, decreased collagen synthesis.
Neurological symptoms	Decreased synthesis of many neurotransmitters.
Viral infections or poor immunity	Protease inhibitor (at high zinc dose) e.g. inhibits action of carboxypeptidase A, thermo-lysine, collagenase, angiotensin-converting enzyme, neutral endopeptidases.
Night blindness	Decreased activity of alcohol dehydrogenase in the retina.

CHAPTER 4

Contingent Nutrient Factors

Enzymes and Miscellaneous Factors

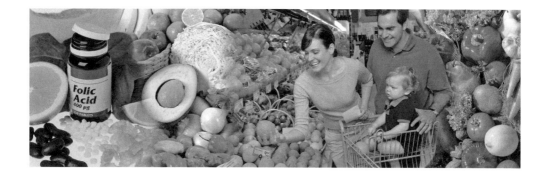

Adenosine

(Purine nucleoside)   Contingent nutrient

SOURCE
Purine rich foods – offal, heart, kidney, brain.

FACTORS INCREASING DEMAND
Central Nervous System (CNS) trauma, epilepsy, tissue ischaemia.

FUNCTIONS FACILITATED
Acts as a chemoprotective agent, acts as a regulatory molecule by binding G-protein associated cell surface receptors A1, A2, A3, acts as purinergic inhibitory neurotransmitter substances, acts as a neuroprotective agent, acts as a vasodilator in all arterioles except those of the kidney, component of cellular energy molecules in ATP, ADP & AMP; inhibits adrenaline release, inhibits the production of reactive oxygen species, inhibits calcium dependent neurotransmitter releases, inhibits nerve cell firing and neurotransmitter release, particularly of aspartate & glutamate; induces sedation, inhibits platelet aggregation and lipolysis, improves white blood cell count after chemotherapy and radiation, inhibits invasion of neutrophils thus attenuates ischaemic/reperfusion injury; increases coronary blood flow during stress and hypoxia, stimulates VEGF and hence angiogenesis, natural sleep molecule of the brain, it induces sedation and sleep, neuroprotective agent, inhibits both spontaneous and evoked nerve firing, neuromodulator of the central and peripheral nervous system, reduces cellular energy consumption, reduces neuronal excitability, stimulates or down regulates adenyl cyclase, topical application improves wound healing in diabetics, A1 and A2 receptor stimulation induces production of granulocyte colony stimulating factor (G-CSF), which stimulates production of white blood cells; inhibits the action of orexin.

Decreased adenosine activity increases dopamine activity.

THERAPEUTIC USES
Allergic urethritis, Alzheimer's disease, anxiety, arrhythmia, cerebral ischaemia, coronary artery disease, chemotherapy, chronic pain, CNS trauma, depression, epilepsy, headaches, Huntington's disease, insomnia, neurodegenerative disease, opiate withdrawal, Parkinson's disease, porphyria cutanea tarda, poor cellular immunity, poor sleep, radiation exposure, self mutilation behaviour, stroke, tachycardia.

DAILY DOSAGE	
SR	100-400 mg

(Taken sublingually for CNS effects).

Unbound adenosine has a half-life of 10-20 seconds.

Once adenosine binds with its receptor, it has a prolonged half-life of 1-2 hours.

Note: Adenosine deaminase catalyses the conversion of adenosine to inosine, which can increase the production of free radicals and increase ischaemic reperfusion injury.

Inosine is metabolised by hypo-xanthine and in the process produce super oxide anions.

CONTRAINDICATIONS
Gout, metastasis.

DRUG/ NUTRIENT INTERACTIONS

Beta blockers, Theophylline, caffeine, opiates. Theobromine reduces the action of adenosine. **Dipyridamole** potentiates the action of adenosine.

RECEPTOR BINDING

Adenosine binds to four receptors – A1, A2A, A2B, and A3. All are G protein coupled receptors. The primary receptors are A1, A2A.

Adenosine A1 receptor:

Linked to inhibition of adenyl cyclase activity.

Activates synthesis of granulocyte colony stimulating factor (G-CSF).

Mediates the inhibition of transmitter release.

Reduces neuronal activity.

Has high affinity for adenosine.

Inhibited by caffeine, theophylline, and coffee.

Adenosine A2A receptor:

Linked to stimulation of adenyl cyclase activity.

Localised in specific areas of the brain such as the caudate and putamen bodies, olfactory bulb and nucleus accumbens. It is also present in platelets.

Has low affinity for adenosine.

Adenosine A3 receptor:

Stimulation of this receptor with high dose adenosine induces: apoptosis of leukemia HL-60, lymphoma, epidermoid cells and GH3 pituitary cell lines.

Activates G-CSF.

SIDE EFFECTS

May cause flushing, dyspnoea and headaches. Taking coffee may relieve headache.

STRUCTURE OF ADENOSINE

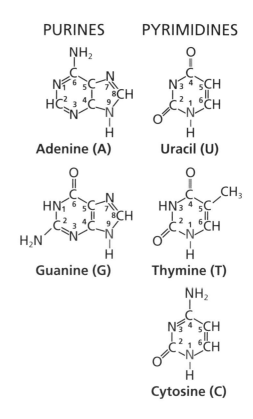

Adenosine is a nucleoside comprised of adenine attached to a ribose (ribofuranose) moiety via a _-N$_9$-glycosidic bond.

PURINES   PYRIMIDINES

Adenine (A)   Uracil (U)

Guanine (G)   Thymine (T)

Cytosine (C)

Alpha-Ketoglutarate

Contingent nutrient

SOURCE
Offal, heart muscle.

FACTORS INCREASING DEMAND
Chronic fatigue, mitochondrial dysfunction due to nitric oxide (NO) excess, strenuous exercise.

FUNCTIONS FACILITATED
Supports mitochondrial function, improves oxygen uptake by mitochondria, competitive inhibitor of glycation, decreases lactate concentration during strenuous exercise, reduces blood ammonia in hepatic cirrhosis, inhibits the generation of high molecular glycated aggregates associated with cataract formation, increases muscle store of glutamine, has an anabolic effect in cancer patients and postoperative patients, improves growth hormone and hormone secretion.

THERAPEUTIC USES
Type I and II diabetes, chronic fatigue, chronic hepatopathy, prevention of diabetic cataracts, strenuous exercise, mitochondrial dysfunction, ophthalmoplegia, inflammation, poor energy, athletes, poor growth in children, conditions of excessive NO production e.g. rheumatoid arthritis and asthma, elevated plasma lactic and pyruvic acid.

DAILY DOSAGE	
SR	1-3 gm/day
For growth promotion:	10-15 gm

SYNERGISTIC NUTRIENTS
Vitamin B_6, leucine, malic acid, magnesium.

DRUG/NUTRIENT INTERACTIONS
Phenformin

STRUCTURE OF ALPHA KETOGLUTARATE

α-**ketoglutarate**, an intermediate in the Krebs cycle, is interconvertible by transamination to glutamic acid.

Betaine Hydrochloride

(24% hydrochloric acid, 76% betaine)

SOURCE

Betaine – astragalus, Echinacea, beetroot, broccoli, spinach, wheat flour.

FUNCTIONS FACILITATED

Assists digestion by increasing hydrochloric acid in the stomach, destroys detrimental bacteria in the stomach and small intestine, required for absorption of histidine, beta-carotene, calcium, iron, magnesium, zinc, vitamin B_{12}, enhances absorption of folic acid and vitamin C, HCl facilitates the flow of bile, methyl donor, stimulates conversion of pepsinogen to pepsin, facilitates normal metabolic pathway of tyrosine, protects against bile acid induced apoptosis.

FACTORS INCREASING DEMAND

Aspirin use, high dose niacin supplement use, poor digestion, low hydrochloric acid production, excessive alcohol consumption.

THERAPEUTIC USES

Bloating, gastric reflux, heartburn, hypochlorhydria, homocystinuria, carbon tetrachloride induced nephrotoxicity, cystathione beta synthase deficiency, cholestatic liver disease, niacin hepatotoxicity, non alcoholic steatohepatitis, xerostomia (dry mouth).

DAILY DOSAGE

500-650mg per large meal

TECHNICAL NOTES

SYNERGISTIC NUTRIENTS

Pancreatic enzymes, folic acid, B_{12}, B_6, choline, lecithin.

DRUG/NUTRIENT INTERACTIONS

Metformin, cholestyramine, aspirin.

STRUCTURE OF BETAINE

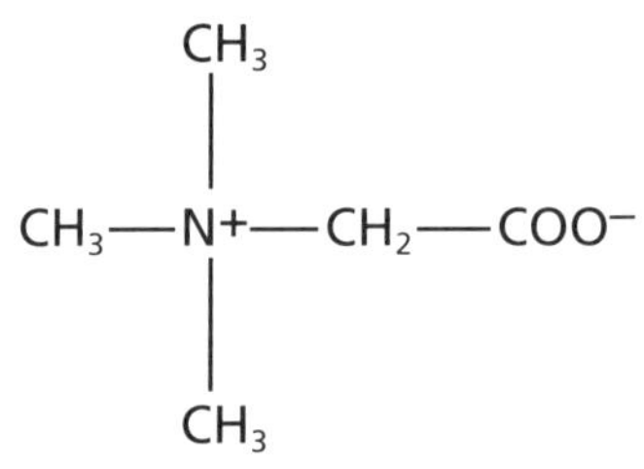

$$CH_3—N^+—CH_2—COO^-$$

with CH_3 groups above and below the nitrogen.

$C_5H_{11}NO_2$: 117.15

Bromelain

SOURCE
Derived from the pineapple plant – Annas cosmosus (Bromeliaceae).

PROCESSING LOSS
Unstable to heat.

FUNCTIONS FACILITATED
Activates proteolytic activity at site of inflammation, anti-inflammatory enzyme, anti-tumour action, accelerates wound healing, anti-metastatic activity, breaks down cholesterol plaques, cardiovascular and circulatory function, fibrinolytic activity, inhibits or modulates the release of inflammatory prostaglandins (PGE_2), immune modulator, induces the production of tumour necrosing factor alpha, interleukin 2 beta, 6 and 8; proteolytic enzyme, increases immuno-toxic effect of monocytes against tumours, modulates bradykinin action, mucolytic activity, prevents platelet aggregation, reduces oedema, reduces the activity of substance P and interferon gamma, regulates MMP activity, removes CD_{44} glycoprotein from lymphocytes.

THERAPEUTIC USES
Angina pectoris, athletic injuries, arthritic stiffness, atherosclerosis, autoimmune disease, bronchiectasis, bronchitis, bronchopneumonia, cholesterol deposits, contusions, enhances the absorption of drugs e.g. flavonoids, glucosamine, antibiotics and tetracycline; haematomas, hypertension, inflammatory disorders of the musculo-skeletal system, inflammatory bowel disease, breast cancer, metastasis associated with platelet aggregation, metastatic cancers, oedema, osteoarthritis, ovarian cancer, pain, pneumonia, post operative tissue reactions and lacerations, painful breasts, pulmonary abscess, pyelonephritis, radiation burns, rheumatoid arthritis, sinusitis, splenectomy, sprains, strains, surgical thrombosis, thrombophlebitis, trauma, wound healing, ulcerative colitis.

DAILY DOSAGE	
SR	150-1600 mg/day or 10-20 mg/kg body wt (1000 mg equiv. 1200 GDU) pH range of activity: pH 4.5-9.8

ADVERSE REACTIONS
Nausea, skin reactions, vomiting, increase in heart rate.

Individuals sensitive to pineapple products should not take this product.

Avoid inhalation of bromelain as it is a strong sensitiser.

SYNERGISTIC NUTRIENTS
Vitamin C, bioflavonoids, quercetin, cysteine, glucosamine, magnesium, pancreatic enzymes.

DRUG/NUTRIENT INTERACTIONS
Warfarin; bromelain promotes its action.
Bromelain increases the absorption of most antibiotics e.g. tetracycline.

Carnitine

Contingent nutrient Acetyl-L-carnitine

SOURCE

Avocado, beef, chicken, fish, milk, liver.

FACTORS INCREASING DEMAND

Adrenal insufficiency, alcohol, athletes, babies fed with soy-based formula, cardiomyopathy, chronic haemodialysis, chronic hypoxia, coeliac disease, deficiency of lysine, methionine, B_3, B_6, C and iron; diabetes, hemodialysis, high fat diets, hyperthyroidism, hypopituitarism, ketosis, limb girdle-muscular dystrophy, muscular dystrophy, myxoedema, new born infants, obesity, premature infants, renal failure, Rett's syndrome, total parenteral nutrition.

FUNCTIONS FACILITATED

Fat metabolism (beta oxidation of fats), gene replication, increases HDL cholesterol, improves neuronal energetics, improve sperm mobility, maximises ATP production in heart muscle, transfers fatty acids across mitochondrial membrane, neuro-protective, peripheral antagonist of thyroid hormone action, modulates intra-mitochondrial acetyl coenzyme A/coenzyme A ratio, facilitates the removal of short chain fatty acids from the mitochondria, enhances physical endurance, increases heart muscle viability after ischaemic injury, utilises ketone bodies, reduces LDL cholesterol.

DEFICIENCY MAY BE ASSOCIATED WITH:

Type-1 lipid storage myopathy, atherosclerosis, cardiomyopathy, CNS dysfunction, cognitive delay, confusion, elevated cholesterol and triglycerides, fasting-hypoglycaemia, fatigue, fatty liver, gastrointestinal dysmotility, heart disease, hyperammonae-mia with muscle ache, hypoprothrombinae-mia, increased fat storage in skeletal muscles, heart and liver; isovaleric acidaemia, lipid storage myopathy, metabolic encephalopathy, methylmalonic-aciduria, muscle weakness and necrosis, myoglobinuria, obesity, propionic aciduria, tiredness.

THERAPEUTIC USES

Abdominal cramps, ADHD, age-related cognitive decline, alcoholism, amenorrhea, angina, AIDS, anorexia, arrhythmia, asthma, athletic performance, cachexia, cancer, cirrhosis, cancer cachexia, cerebral atoxia, chemotherapy-induced neuropathy, chronic fatigue, chronic fatigue syndrome, chronic hepatitis, coeliac disease, congestive and ischaemic heart disease, COPD, cystic fibrosis, depression, diabetes, dialysis patients, diphtheria, Down's syndrome, emphysema, endurance, fatigue, hepatic cancer, HIV patients, hypertension, hypercholesterolemia, hyperthyroidism, hypertriglyceremia, hypoglycaemia, improves sperm mobility, increased appetite, infertility (male), inflammatory myopathies, intermittent claudication, irregular heart beat, ischemic reperfusion surgery, ischaemia, ketosis, kidney disease, kidney dialysis, macular degeneration, mental decline, muscular dystrophy, myocardial infarction, myopathy, obesity, organic aciduria, Parkinson's disease, peripheral heart disease, peripheral neuropathy (secondary trauma), peyronie's disease, poor circulation, pre-neoplastic lesions, rashes, Rett's syndrome, Reye's syndrome, ventricular fibrillation, vomiting, tumours, vegetarians.

DAILY DOSAGE	
RDA	None given (~ 400 mg/day)
SR	400-6000 mg

15-65% of the carnitine is absorbed (absorption can be variable).

50-200 mg/kg body weight is required for some lipid storage disease.

Glucose reduces acetyl-L-carnitine uptake across the blood brain barrier.

EFFECTS OF OVERDOSAGE AND TOXICITY

Diarrhoea, irritability, ketosis, lethargy, personality changes, fish odour syndrome.

DRUG/NUTRIENT INTERACTIONS

Valproic acid, Zidovudine (AZT), Adriamycin, Cefotetan, Pivoxil.

STRUCTURE OF CARNITINE

3-carboxy-2-hydroxy-N,N,N-trimethyl-1-propanaminium

Acetyl-L-Carnitine

FUNCTIONS FACILITATED

Counter-acts the age related reduction in glucocorticoid receptors, prevents the phosphorylation of Tau protein, acetylates alpha and beta proteins thus preventing the formation of amyloid sheets, induces haeme oxygenase 1, which increases carbon monoxide (CO) production and up-regulates HSP60; increases the expression of redox sensitive transcription factor NrF2 in the nucleus of cells, up-regulates nerve growth factor; modulates brain energy and phospholipid metabolism, modulates synaptic morphology and synaptic transmission of multiple neurotransmitters; involved in the acetylation of Nh_2 and − OH functional groups in amino acids.

THERAPEUTIC USES

ADHD, ageing, aged related memory loss, Alzheimer's disease, axonal peripheral neuropathy associated with oxaliplatin and HIV drug treatment, epilepsy, geriatric depression, hepatic coma, ischaemic stress, methamphetamine addiction during the withdrawal phase; kidney failure, neurodegeneration, senile depression, stress, sympathetic dominance.

DAILY DOSAGE	
RDA	None given (~ 400 mg/day)
SR	400-6000 mg

OVERDOSAGE

Alzheimers patients may become more aggressive.

Some epilepsy patients may experience more seizures.

TECHNICAL NOTES

SYNERGISTIC NUTRIENTS

Vitamin B_3, B_5, B_6, B_{12}, C, folic acid, lysine, iron, magnesium, methionine, phosphatidylserine, potassium.

DRUG/NUTRIENT INTERACTIONS

Oxaliplatin; Nucleoside analogues didanosine (ddl), zalcitabine (ddC), and stavudine (d4T) use in the treatment of HIV, induce acetylcarnitine deficiency.

ENZYME SYSTEMS INVOLVED

Carnitine acyl-transferase

Heme oxygenase 1

Acetyl-L-carnitine is also known as acetyl-carnitine, L-acetycarnitine, acetylcarnitine, acetyl levocarnitine, ALC and ALCAR.

STRUCTURE OF ACETYL-L-CARNITINE

$$(CH_3)_3N^+ — CH_2 \sim CH —— CH_2 —COO^-$$

with the branch:
O
CCH₃ (CCH_3)
O

Acetyl-L-carnitine is also known as acetyl-carnitine, L-acetycarnitine, acetylcarnitine, acetyl levocarnitine, ALC and ALCAR.

Carnosine

Beta-alanyl-L histidine   Contingent nutrient

SOURCE

Muscle meats, brain, heart, fish.

FACTORS INCREASING DEMAND

Muscle injury, strenuous exercise, cancer, diabetes, hyperglycaemia.

FUNCTIONS FACILITATED

Activates cellular Na+K+ATPase, acts as an intracellular pH buffer in muscle, acts as a histidine reserve, antioxidant activity, protects against DNA oxidation, anti-ischaemic effects, blocks the growth of beta amyloid peptide aggregates, chelates heavy metals, enhances prefrontal cortex function, ergogenic aid, improves cardiac contractibility, improves autistic behaviour; inactivates and/or disposes aged proteins by reacting with them to produce lipofuscin or by promoting proteolysis of these proteins; increases language comprehension, inhibits lipid peroxidation and protein and LDL cholesterol oxidation, modulates the activity of brain tyrosine, protects against the hydroxyl radical, prevents protein glycation reactions, sensitises cellular calcium channels to their activators, reduces glycation of protein due to ribose and fructose. Protects the body from glycation reactions, chelates heavy metals Pb, Hg, Ni, Cu & Zn. Facilitates nitric oxidise production in endothelial cells, neuroprotective, maintains brain-glutathione levels, reduced ROS production in ischemic tissue, decreases blood sugar levels. Protects cells from oxidation-induced stress damage, extends life of cultured cells, rejuvenates senescent cells, inhibits toxic effects of amyloid peptides (amyloid beta), reduces the onsets of eyesight failure, prevents senile cataracts & reduces age-related diseases.

THERAPEUTIC USES

Acute renal failure, ageing, athletes, Alzheimer's disease, autistic spectrum disorder, cancer patients, cerebral ischemia, diabetes, diabetic cataracts, diabetic neuropathy, gentamicin-induced nephrotoxicity, heart failure, hypertension, hyperglycaemia, ischemic reperfusion injury, liver disease, loss of smell, neurodegenerative disorders, polymyositis, recovery from muscle injury, reduces hyperglycaemic toxicity, stroke, sepsis, trauma, wound healing.

DAILY DOSAGE	
SR	100-4000 mg

Note: Dosages >1000 mg in hyperactive or manic autistic patients may show signs of: overstimulation, hyperactivity, irritability and insomnia.

SYNERGISTIC NUTRIENTS

Taurine, histidine, alanine, lipoic acid, zinc, vitamin E.

STRUCTURE OF CARNOSINE AND HOMOCARNOSINE

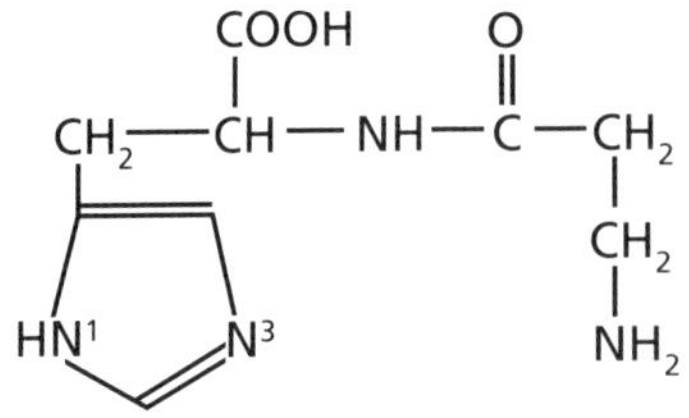

β-alanyl-L-histidine
$C_{11}H_{16}N_4O_4$
Carnosine is a naturally-occurring multifunctional dipeptide formed from the chemical combination of amino acids beta-alanine and histidine.

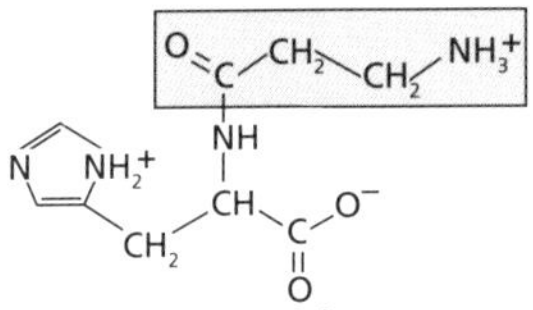

Carnosine

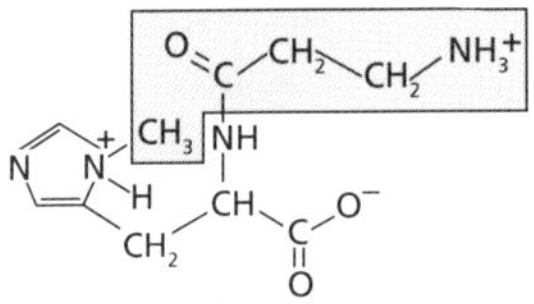

Anserine

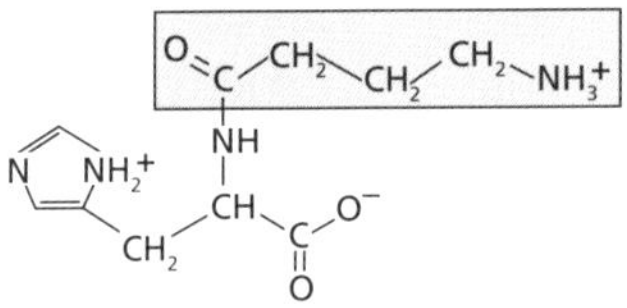

Homocarnosine

Carnosine-like Molecules

Homocarnosine (gamma-aminobutyryl-L-histidine) is a dipeptide composed of the amino acids Gamma-aminobutyric Acid (GABA, the primary inhibitor brain neurotransmitter) and L-histidine. Carnosine and homocarnosine are both produced by the same ATP-driven enzyme, **carnosine synthetase**, and both molecules exhibit very similar properties. The concentration of homocarnosine in the human brain, however, is about 100 times that of carnosine. It is manufactured by glial cells (oligodendrocytes) except in the olfactory bulb, where it is synthesized by neurons. The highest brain homocarnosine concentrations are found in the substantia nigra, dentate gyrus and olfactory bulb, as well as in the cerebrospinal fluid.

Co enzyme Q$_{10}$

(Ubiquinone, Ubidecarenone, CoQ$_{10}$)

FACTORS INCREASING DEMAND

Antidepressants, beta-blocker drugs, cancer, candida infections, chemotherapy, cholesterol lowering drugs, diabetes, ageing, HIV infection, ischaemic heart disease, muscular dystrophies, Parkinson's disease, radiation.

FUNCTIONS FACILITATED

Acts as a lipid antioxidant, cofactor in several metabolic pathways particularly oxidative respiration, lowers blood pressure, improves the energetics of the immune cellular system, increases IgG levels in response to infection, prevents cellular depletion of ATP, reduces aldosterone secretion and inhibits the effects of angiotensin, reduces blood viscosity and fibrinogen levels, reduces low density lipoprotein (LDL) peroxidation during oxidative stress, improves cardiac bioenergetics, protects ATPase protein from oxidation, normalises cancer cells, spares vitamin E, stabilisers myocardial calcium ion channels, strengthens the heart.

CoQ$_{10}$ is a cofactor in oxidative phosphorylation through the electron transport chain. It transfers electrons from flavo-proteins to cytochromes. Putative modulator of miRNA- 146, thus reducing inflammation.

DEFICIENCY MAY CAUSE OR BE ASSOCIATED WITH:

Angina, cardiomyopathy, diabetes, fatigue, heart disease, heart failure, muscular dystrophy, infection, periodontal disease.

THERAPEUTIC USES

Acute hearing loss, AIDS, Alzheimer's disease, angina; anthracycline chemotherapy drug (doxorubicin) therapy arrhythmia, atherosclerosis, bronchial asthma, cachexia, cancer (breast, lung, prostate, pancreatic, cervical), chronic inflammation, congestive heart failure, chronic fatigue, chronic obstructive pulmonary disease (COPD), chronic malnutrition, dilated cardiomyopathy, diabetes, dyspermia, fatigue, Friedreich's ataxia, gastric ulcers, gingivitis, haemorrhagic shock, heart failure, HIV infection, hypercholesterolaemia, hypertension, hyperthyroidism, hypoxia, ischaemic heart disease, medical drug use – statins, mitochondrial encephalomyopathies, morbid obesity, muscular dystrophy, Parkinson's disease, periodontal disease, radiation, radiation pneumonitis infection, retinitis pigmentosa, sensory neuropathy, toxin induced cardiotoxicity.

DOSAGE	
SR	90-600 mg

SIDE EFFECTS

Diarrhoea, dizziness, epigastric discomfort, occasional nausea (over 250mg).

DRUG/NUTRIENT INTERACTIONS

Decreases CoQ10 absorption:
 Orlistat

Decrease formation of CoQ10 in the body:
 Beta-blockers –atenolol, esmolol, betaxolol, penbutolol, carteolol, bisoprolol, pindolol, metoprolol, timolol, sotalol, acebutolol, nadolol, propranolol, labetalol, carvedilol, levobunolol, levobetaxolol, metipranolol
 HMG-CoA reductase inhibitors – atorvastatin, fluvastatin, lovastatin, pravastatin, simvastatin
 Phenothiazines – chlorpromazine, thioridazine, fluphenazine, trifluoperazine, mesoridazine, prochlorperazine, perphenazine, promethazine
 Tricyclic antidepressants – amitriptyline, amoxapine, clomipramine, desipramine, doxepin, imipramine, nortriptyline, protryptiline, trimipramine
 Biguanides – metformin
 Thiazide diuretics – hydrochlorothiazide, chlorothiazide, indapamide, metolazone, chlorthalidone, hydroflumethiazide, polythiazide, trichlormethiazide, benzthiazide, methyclothiazide, bendroflumethiazide
 Clonidine, Haloperidol, Hydralazine, Methyldopa

Decrease body levels of CoQ10:
 Gemfibrozil

 Sulfonylureas – glyburide, glipizide, glimepiride, tolbutamide, tolazamide, acetohexamide, chlorpropamide

 Adriamycin, doxorubicin, glaucoma drugs

TECHNICAL NOTES

SYNERGISTIC NUTRIENTS

R-lipoic acid, vitamin E, vitamin C, selenium, glutathione.

For synthesis of CoQ_{10} – tyrosine, folate, vitamins B_2, B_3, B_5, B_6, B_{12} and C.

TARGET TISSUES

Heart, liver, kidney, pancreas.

STRUCTURE OF COENZYME Q10

Coenzyme Q$_{10}$

Ubiquinol (CoQH$_2$)

Semiquinone radical (CoQH$\cdot$)

Ubiquinone (CoQ)

CoQ_{10} (2, 3-dimethoxy-5-methylbenzoquinone) is a fat-soluble quinone ring attached to 10 isoprene side units, structurally similar to vitamin K. In humans, CoQ_{10} is found in relatively higher concentrations in cells with high-energy requirements such as: heart, liver, muscle, and pancreas. Normal blood levels range from 0.7-1.0 µg/ml. Human cells synthesize CoQ_{10} from the amino acid tyrosine, in an eight-step aromatic pathway, requiring adequate levels of vitamins such as folic acid, niacin, riboflavin, and pyridoxine. A deficiency in any of these nutrients would result in a deficiency in CoQ_{10}.

Creatine

Alpha-methyl guanidino acetic acid   N-(aminoiminomethyl)-N-methyl glycine
Contingent nutrient

SOURCE
Muscle meats.

FACTORS INCREASING DEMAND
Cardiac surgery, high intensity exercises, vegetarian diets.

FUNCTIONS FACILITATED
Attenuates corticosteroid induced muscle wasting, Improves bioenergetics of heart muscle, improves muscle protein synthesis, improves working memory and general intelligence, improves mitochondrial bioenergetics, improves neurological protection against ischaemia and oxidant insult, improves training capacity, reduces muscle lactate during exercise.

Precursor of phosphocreatine – a high energy intermediate.

- Phosphocreatine inhibits enzymes in the glycolytic pathway, including: glyceraldehyde-3-phosphate dehydrogenase, phosphofructo-kinase and pyruvate kinase.

Twelve weeks of resistance training combined with creatine supplementation increases muscle fibre diameter by 35% in both Type 1 and 2 muscle fibres in men vs. 6-15% in placebo-supplemented resistance trained subjects.

THERAPEUTIC USES
Amyotrophic lateral sclerosis; arginine: glycine aminidinotransferase (AGAT), S-adenosyl-L-methionine: N-guanidino-acetate methyltransferase (GAMT) deficiency; basal cell carcinoma, body builders, brain trauma, angiomas, cancer, cardiac surgery, congestive heart failure, cramps associated with haemodialysis, Duchenne muscular dystrophy, gyrate atrophy (vision loss due to muscle weakness), hepatic disease, high intensity exercise, Huntington's disease, leukaemia, mitochondrial cytopathies, muscle diseases, muscle strengthening, neuro-degenerative disease, Parkinson's disease, rheumatoid arthritis, sprint athletes, steroid induced myopathy.

TARGET ORGANS
Skeletal muscle, cardiac tissue, smooth muscle, brain, kidney, sperm.

DAILY DOSAGE	
SR	1-5 g/day

Acute loading for sport: 20gm for two days or 5 gm for five days in divided doses.

Note: About 1 to 2 grams of creatine are biosynthesized daily and another 1 to 2 grams are obtained from diet.

Creatine is contraindicated in those with renal failure and renal disorders such as nephrotic syndrome.

SYNERGISTIC NUTRIENTS
Arginine, glycine, methionine, leucine, carbohydrate loading, chromium.

SIDE EFFECTS
Weight gain, cramps, dehydration, diarrhoea, dizziness.

Alpha-methylguanidino acetic acid

Creatine is synthesized in the kidney, liver and pancreas from three different amino acids: arginine, glycine, and methionine. It is converted into creatinine before elimination by the kidneys.

Dietary Fibre

ACTIVE INGREDIENTS
Cellulose, gums, hemicellulose, lignin, mucilage, pectin substances, plant sterols, saponins.

SOURCE
Apple pectin, blueberries, bran, oat meal, couscous, cucumbers, celery, pears, psyllium seeds, guar gums, raw salad vegetables, sorghum, wholegrain cereals, zucchini.

PROCESSING LOSSES
Food processing and refining of cereal grains results in appreciable loss.

FACTORS INCREASING DEMAND
Colon cancer, constipation, coronary artery disease, diabetes, diarrhoea, diverticulitis, gallstones, haemorrhoids, hypercholesterolaemia, obesity.

FUNCTIONS FACILITATED
Guar gum and pectin
Binds cholesterol, gives satiety effects, promotes optimum colonic environment for gut bacteria, regulates glucose absorption from the gut.

Psyllium, bran
Binds cholesterol, bowel detoxification, gives bulk to stool, improves transit time through the bowel, reduces pressure in the bowel.

Pectin
Broken down by gut bacteria to oligosaccharide, which inhibits cancer cells from adhering to vascular wall.

Lignans (Present in flaxseed meal)
Reduces hormone sensitive cancers – prostate and breast cancer, by binding unconjugated sex hormones.

Inhibits or down-regulates the enzyme aromatase (enzyme involved in sex hormone synthesis).

Colonic fermentation of fibre produces acetic, butyric and propionic acid. Butyric acid normalises abnormal colonocytes and reduces the risk of colon cancer.

DEFICIENCY SYMPTOMS
Constipation, diverticular disease, gall bladder disease, heart disease.

THERAPEUTIC USES
Cancer prevention, constipation, coronary artery disease, diabetes, diarrhoea, diverticulitis, elevated blood cholesterol and triglycerides, gall stones, haemorrhoids, heart disease, hiatus hernia, irritable bowel syndrome, weight reduction.

DAILY DOSAGE	
RDA	>20 gm
SR	12-20 gm

SYNERGISTIC NUTRIENTS
Lactobacillus acidophilus, Bifidobacterium species, DHA/EPA, water.

DRUG/NUTRIENT INTERACTIONS
Oral Medications
In general, **fibre supplements** should probably be taken at least 2 hours apart from doses of prescription drugs. The ingestion of large quantities of fiber could possibly change the absorption of numerous drugs from the intestinal tract. eg. Lovastatin, Digoxin, lithium
Soluble fibers affect blood glucose and insulin levels, which could alter the effects of anti-diabetic medications and possibly the dose needed for treatment. e.g.
Diabetic/Hypoglycemic medications – Insulin, glyburide, glipizide, metformin, rosiglitazone, pioglitazone, glimepiride, tolbutamide, tolazamide, acarbose, acetohexamide, chlorpropamide, miglitol, repaglinide, nateglinide.

Dimethyl Glycine

Contingent nutrient

SOURCE
Brewer's yeast, brown rice, organ meats, seeds, wholegrain cereals.

FACTORS INCREASING DEMAND
Alcohol, athletic performance, coffee, diabetes, heart failure, lung diseases.

FUNCTIONS FACILITATED
Increases glycogen, creatine phosphate, phospholipid and total lipid content in cardiac and skeletal muscle; increases body's tolerance to hypoxia, increases oxygen uptake by tissues, improves circulation, may act as precursor to the neurotransmitter glycine, possible methyl donor, reduces lactate production in exercise, stimulates cytochrome oxidase and oxidative-phosphorylating capacities.

DEFICIENCY MAY CAUSE OR BE ASSOCIATED WITH:
None reported.

THERAPEUTIC USES
Angina, atherosclerosis, autism, ADHD, cardio-pulmonary insufficiency, diabetes, eczema, emphysema, epilepsy, headaches, heart disease, liver disease, intermittent claudication, jaundice, poor circulation, shortness of breath, stroke, viral hepatitis.

DAILY DOSAGE	
RDA	50 mg (Russian standard)
SR	50-300 mg

EFFECTS OF OVERDOSAGE AND TOXICITY
Drowsiness, mild flushing of skin.

TECHNICAL NOTES

SYNERGISTIC NUTRIENTS
Vitamin C, betaine, choline, methionine.

DRUG/NUTRIENT INTERACTIONS
5-Fluorouracil, corticosteroids, Digoxin, Strophanthin, sulpha drugs.

STRUCTURE OF DIMETHYL GLYCINE

Dimethylglycine (N,N-Dimethylglycine)

DMG is metabolized in the liver to monomethylglycine or sarcosine which, in turn, is converted to glycine.

Dimethylglycine dehydrogenase, a flavoprotein, is the enzyme that catalyses the oxidative demethylation of DMG to sarcosine. The methyl group produced in this reaction returns to the one carbon pool at the level of N^{10}-hydroxymethyl-tetrahydrofolic acid.

DMG itself is formed from trimethylglycine or betaine. DMG that is not metabolized in the liver is transported by the circulatory system to various tissues in the body.

D-Glucaric Acid

SOURCE
Oranges (4.5mg/100gm), broccoli, potato (1.12-1.73 mg/100gm).

FACTORS INCREASING DEMAND
Alcohol ingestion, chemical exposure, kanamycin (antibiotic), oestrogen excess, smokers.

FUNCTIONS FACILITATED
Inhibits beta glucuronidase activity in serum and liver, lung and intestinal microsomes; inhibition of this enzyme has a marked antiproliferative effect on breast tissue, inhibits chemical carcinogen-induced mammary tumours, detoxifies chemicals, increases the metabolism of oestrogen by preventing the deconjugation of the oestrogen-glucuronic complex by beta glucuronidase.

THERAPEUTIC USES
Bowel cancer, breast cancer, chemical exposure e.g. benzo (a) pyrene and plastics, oestrogen excess, nephrotoxicity due to kanamycin.

DAILY DOSAGE	
SR	400-6000 mg/day

SYNERGISTIC NUTRIENTS
Retinoids, vitamin A.

STRUCTURE OF GLUCARIC ACID

5-Dehydro-4-deoxy-D-glucarate

D-mannose

SOURCE

Blackcurrants, cranberry, goose berries, red currants, aloe vera, soy beans, capsicums, cabbages, eggplants, tomatoes, turnips.

FUNCTIONS FACILITATED

Inhibits bacterial (gram positive bacteria) adherence to mucosal surfaces, prevents E. coli from adhering to the walls of bladder and urinary tract, prevention of urinary tract infections.

THERAPEUTIC USES

Cystitis, urinary tract infections, phosphomannose isomerase deficiency (PMI), cystic fibrosis, glycoprotein syndrome 1b.

DAILY DOSAGE	
SR	1500-5000mg every four to six hours

TECHNICAL NOTES

SYNERGISTIC NUTRIENTS

L-fructose, D-arabinose

STRUCTURE OF D- MANNOSE

Mannose is a sugar monomer of the hexose series of carbohydrates.

Mannose differs from D-glucose by inversion of the C2 chiral centre. This apparently simple change leads to the drastically different chemistry of the two hexoses.

Fructo-oligosaccharides (FOS)

(Inulin – fermentable fibres)

SOURCE

Bananas, rye, oats, chicory root, burdock, leaks, onions, garlic, tomatoes, asparagus.

FUNCTIONS FACILITATED

Decreases intestinal pH, enhances liver function, enhances the production of softer bowel motions, facilitates endogenous production of butyric acid, increases faecal lactobacillus and enterobacteria, increases faecal mucin excretion, provides nourishment for beneficial bacteria in the bowel, utilised in the production of bifidobacterium and lactobacillus bacteria.

THERAPEUTIC USES

Antibiotic overuse, candidiasis, colon cancer, constipation, diarrhoea, irritable bowel syndrome, leaky gut syndrome, gut dysbiosis,

DAILY DOSAGE	
SR	1-4g/day

TECHNICAL NOTES

SYNERGISTIC NUTRIENTS

Lactobacillus acidophilus, fibre, slippery elm, glutamine, DHA/EPA.

STRUCTURE OF FRUCTO-OLIGOSACCHARIDES

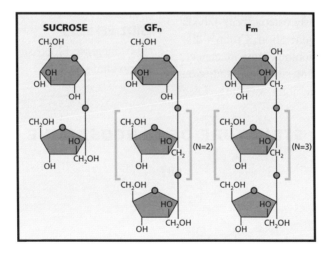

Fructo-oligosaccharides are low molecular weight carbohydrates.

Structurally they are a mixture of polymers (chain repeats of the same unit molecule) and oligomers (chains composed of different molecular units), comprising branching chains of between 10 and 60 units of fructose.

Fructo-oligosaccharides are water soluble, being non viscous 'fructans' and have a low water retention capacity.

As they are not broken down significantly by the digestive processes in the stomach and small intestine, they are classified as dietary fibre.

Glucosamine

Contingent nutrient

SOURCE
Synthesized in the body from glucose; shark cartilage, tracheal cartilage.

FUNCTIONS FACILITATED
Anti-viral activity, liver detoxification, major component of the protective mucous lining of the stomach, major precursor in the synthesis of the mucopolysaccharides (glycoproteins) and proteoglycans found in ground substance and connective tissue, normalises cartilage metabolism, produced by all cells in the body, increases the synthesis of leptin in skeletal and fatty tissue, increases leptin production.

THERAPEUTIC USES
Arthritis (particularly osteoarthritis), back pain, cartilage degeneration, Crohn's disease, enhances chemotherapy in cancer, gastric ulceration, interstitial and radiation cystitis, joint pain, joint swelling, knee damage, liver problems, leaky gut syndrome, post menopausal osteoporosis, poor bone healing, restricted movement, ulcerative colitis.

DAILY DOSAGE

DAILY DOSAGE	
SR	600-3000 mg/day

DRUG/NUTRIENT INTERACTIONS
Many non-steroidal anti-inflammatory drugs inhibit the synthesis of glucosamine and its conversion to mucopolysaccharides e.g. **aspirin, brufen, indomethacin, NSAIDs.**

SYNERGISTIC NUTRIENTS
Vitamin A, manganese, chondroitin sulfate.

SIDE EFFECTS
May increase blood sugar levels if given intravenously.

STRUCTURE OF GLUCOSAMINE

Alpha-D-glucosamine

Glycosaminoglycans or **GAGs** contain derivatives of glucosamine or galactosamine.

Glucosamine derivatives are found in hyaluronic acid, keratan sulfate and heparan sulfate.

Chondroitin sulfate contains derivatives of galactosamine.

N-Acetyl-Glucosamine (NAG)

Contingent nutrient

FUNCTIONS FACILITATED

Makes up the GAG barrier of digestive tract mucous lining, supports gastrointestinal function by enhancing mucosal integrity, component of the glycocalyx coat – a layer of carbohydrate and protein, complexed together, and anchored to the out surface of cell membranes; involved in cell to cell attachment, bulks up and strengthens connective tissue, regulates immune cell activity in the joint. Binds cell surface of T helper cells and reduces the "stay alive signal" produced by T helper cells and thus reduces the activity of activated white blood cells.

THERAPEUTIC USES

Alcoholics, atherosclerosis, chronic inflammation, gut ulceration, inflammatory bowel disease, inflamed joints, osteoarthritis.

DAILY DOSAGE	
SR	1-6g/day

STRUCTURE OF N-ACETYL-GLUCOSAMINE

Glutathione

(GSH)   Tripeptide containing cysteine, glutamic acid and glycine.
Y – glutamyl cysteinyl glycine   Contingent Nutrient

SOURCE

Asparagus, avocado, eggs, garlic, plant and animal tissue, walnut, whey protein.

Cysteine and n-acetyl cysteine supplementation increases GSH.

FACTORS INCREASING DEMAND

Alcohol, aspirin intake, asthma, copper deficiency, Down's syndrome, elderly, excessive exercise, excessive intake of unsaturated fat, heavy metal exposure, hyperglycaemia, immune dysfunction, low protein intake, oral contraceptives, oxidative stress, pollution, rheumatoid arthritis, smoking, ulcers.

FUNCTIONS FACILITATED

Acts as an extracellular antioxidant, antitoxin, boosts immunity, deactivator of free radicals, immune regulation, inhibits activation of nuclear factor Kappa-β (NFK-β), inhibits lipid peroxidation, maintains the essential thiol structure of proteins, provides a reservoir for cysteine, modulates critical cellular processes such as DNA synthesis, microtubular related processes and immune function; protects intestinal endothelial cells against oxidative stress, protects mitochondrial function, prostaglandin synthesis, protects the integrity of red blood cells, reduces replication of HIV virus, vanadium metabolism, detoxifies DDT, epoxides in glue and resins, aflatoxin, xenobiotics and alkylating carcinogens, recycles vitamins E and C, thus maintaining their antioxidant properties.

DEFICIENCY MAY CAUSE OR BE ASSOCIATED WITH:

High incidences of cancer and heart disease, chemical sensitivity, immune dysfunction, increased free radical damage, increases rate of cellular apoptosis, mental deterioration, oxidative stress, poor balance and coordination, premature ageing, lack of balance and co-ordination, lack of body synthesis which leads to an increased risk of chronic degenerative disease e.g. accelerated ageing, lactation failure; tremors.

THERAPEUTIC USES

Ageing, AIDS, aflatoxin exposure, alcoholics, arthritis, asthma, aspirin and phenacetin overdose, atherosclerosis, benzene exposure, cachexia, cancer, chemically sensitive individuals, Crohn's disease, cigarette smoke exposure, diabetes, Down's syndrome, leaky gut, heart disease, heavy metal toxicity, hepatitis, HIV infections, hypertension, hyperbaric oxygen treatment, idiopathic pulmonary fibrosis, impaired liver function, inflammation, irritable bowel, leukoplakia, neurodegenerative disease, oral cancer, Parkinson's disease, poor immunity, radiation therapy, respiratory distress syndrome, ulcerative colitis, urinary tract infection, viral infections, viral induced nutrient deficiency disease.

DAILY DOSAGE	
SR	100-500 mg

TECHNICAL NOTES

SYNERGISTIC NUTRIENTS

Vitamin A, B$_2$, B$_6$, C, E, cysteine, glutamic acid, glycine, lipoic acid, magnesium, methionine, n-acetyl-cysteine, s-adenosyl methionine, selenium, manganese, zinc.

DRUGS INCREASING DEMAND

Alcohol, cisplatin, cycloheximide, cyclophosphamide, dexamethasone, paracetamol, phenacetin.

STRUCTURE OF GLUTATHIONE

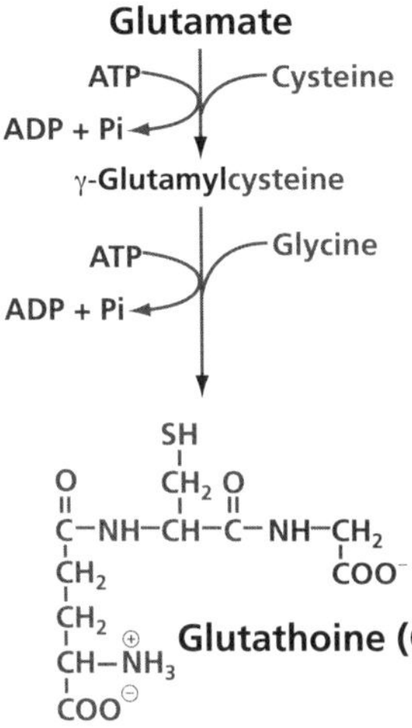

Glutamate

ATP⟶ ⟵ Cysteine

ADP + Pi ⟵

↓

γ-**Glutamyl**cysteine

ATP⟶ ⟵ Glycine

ADP + Pi ⟵

↓

SH
|
CH$_2$
|
O   O
‖   ‖
C–NH–CH–C–NH–CH$_2$
| |
CH$_2$ COO$^-$
|
CH$_2$
|
CH–$\overset{\oplus}{N}$H$_3$ **Glutathoine (GSH)**
|
COO$^\ominus$

$\overset{\oplus}{N}$H$_3$
|
$^\ominus$OOC–CH$_3$
|
CH$_2$
|
CH$_2$
|
O=C
|
NH
|
CH–CH$_2$–S—S—CH$_2$–CH
|
O=C
|
NH
|
CH$_2$
|
COO$^\ominus$

COO$^\ominus$
|
CH$_2$
|
NH
|
C=O
|
CH$_2$
|
C=O
|
CH$_2$
|
CH$_2$
|
CH–COO$^\ominus$
|
$\overset{\oplus}{N}$H$_3$

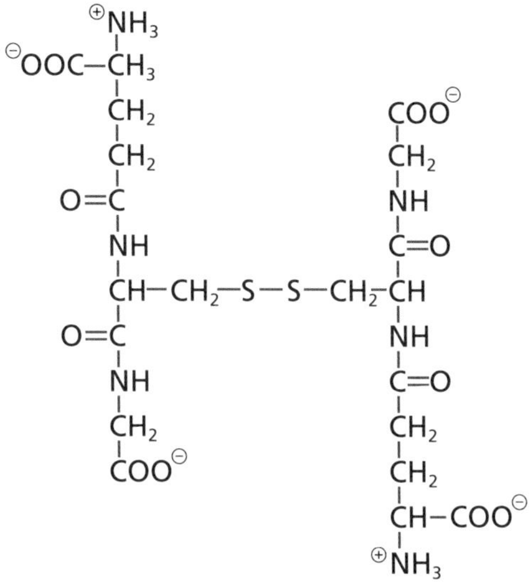

Glutathione disulfide (GSSG)

Glutathione (abbreviated GSH) is a tripeptide composed of glutamate, cysteine and glycine.

Indole 3 Carbinol

I3C

SOURCES

Broccoli, cabbage, cauliflower, kale, Brussels sprouts.

FUNCTIONS FACILITATED

Antioxidant, blocks estrogen receptor sites on the membranes of breast and other cells, thereby reducing the risk of breast and cervical cancer; decreases carcinogen activation by inhibition of phase 1 detoxifying enzymes, counteracts dietary carcinogens, maintains integrity of p53 tumour suppressor gene, helps to prevent breast cancer by stimulating the conversion of oestrogen to 2-hydroxyestrone, inhibits conversion of estrone to 16-hydroxyestrone, facilitates glucuronidation, protects against reactive oxygen species, induces phase II detoxifying enzymes, inhibits P-glycoprotein transport, inhibits STATS activation, increases the expression of interferon gamma receptor 1, induces apoptosis, inhibits MUC1 transmembrane glycoprotein which is over expressed in many cancers, stimulates endogenous production of glutathione in the liver, reduces the ability of some heterocyclic aromatic amines to initiate DNA damage, stimulates the conversion of estrone to 2-hydroxyestrone, slows tumour growth.

THERAPEUTIC USES

Cancer prevention, breast cancer, prostate cancer, cervical dysplasia, liver protection, oestrogen sensitive cancers, respiratory papillomatosis, multi-drug resistant tumours.

DAILY DOSAGE	
SR	400-800mg/day or 5-7mg/kg of body weight

TECHNICAL NOTES

SYNERGISTIC NUTRIENTS

Quercetin, CLA, selenium, genistein, vitamin C

DRUG/NUTRIENT INTERACTIONS
Oral contraceptive pills, oestrogen containing drugs, enhance the effects of tamoxifen.

STRUCTURE OF INDOLE-3-CARBINOL

3-indolemethanol **Formula: $C_9H_9N_O$**

Inositol

Myoinositol, cis-1,2,3,5, trans-4,6, cyclohexanehexol
Contingent nutrient

SOURCE

Bacterial synthesis in the gut, beans, brewers yeast, cantaloupe, citrus fruit, corn, grains, lecithin, lentils, nuts, organ meats, pork, seeds, veal.

FACTORS INCREASING DEMAND

Blood pressure, chronic renal failure, diabetes, high blood cholesterol, impaired kidney function, lactation, premature infants, stress, uraemia, respiratory distress syndrome, chronic renal failure.

FUNCTIONS FACILITATED

Precursor of the second messenger system in intracellular communication, component of cell membranes, facilitates synthesis of arachidonic acid, helps absorb zinc, helps cytoskeleton assembly, lowers cortisol and reduces HPA stress response, liver function, modulates serotonin activity, myelin synthesis, RNA synthesis, saturated fat absorption from intestine, promotes endothelial cell growth, regulates intracellular calcium, regulates cell surface phenomena such as binding of hormones and electrical transfer in neural tissue, stimulates lung surfactant production.

Inositol is a key intermediate of the phosphatidyl – inositol cycle, a second messenger system used by several noradrenergic, serotonergic and cholinergic receptors (helps to restore their function).

Inositol is a component of inositides.

Inositides are a diverse and multifunctional group of cellular components, which have in common myo-inositol as part of their chemical structure. Inositides can be classified into two very different basic types, whose metabolism and functions are mostly separate: the inositol lipids and inositol phosphates.

(1) Inositol lipids – Central to most inositide metabolism and function is the inositol lipid, phosphatidylinositol 4,5-bisphosphate (PIP2). It is the precursor for at least three second messengers, inositol 1,4,5-trisphosphate (IP3), diacylglycerol, and phosphatidylinositol 3,4,5-trisphosphate, and itself plays an important regulatory role in, for example, cytoskeletal function.

(2) Inositol phosphates – Once IP3 is generated in the cytosol, it is rapidly metabolised by two routes: by dephosphorylation (ultimately to inositol) and by phosphorylation to inositol 1,3,4,5-tetrabisphosphate (IP4).

DEFICIENCY MAY CAUSE OR BE ASSOCIATED WITH:

Alopecia, cataracts, constipation, eczema, eye problems, hypercholesterolaemia, impaired lipid transport, lipodystrophies, liver lipid accumulation and secretion, platelet aggregation, tardive dyskinesia.

THERAPEUTIC USES

Alcoholism, agyrophobia, anxiety, atherosclerosis, bulimia, bipolar disorder, cataracts, constipation, depression, diabetes, diabetic cataract, hair loss, heart disease, high blood cholesterol, insomnia, ketosis, lactation, premature infants, prevention of neural tube defects, panic disorder, post-traumatic stress disorder, obsessive compulsive disorder, sciatica, social phobia, uraemia.

DAILY DOSAGE	
RDA	500-1000 mg
SR	750-13,000 mg

Neonates with respiratory distress – 80mg/kg body weight.

Inositol needs to be taken over a prolonged period to get therapeutic effect.

EFFECTS OF OVERDOSAGE AND TOXICITY	
>0.5g/kg body weight	diarrhoea, increase excretion of creatine.

DRUG/NUTRIENT INTERACTIONS

Aminoglycosides, antibiotics, cyclosporin, chlortetracycline, doxycycline, d-glucose excess, fluoroquinolones, lithium, macrolide, minocycline, penicillin, sulfonamides, tetracycline, trimethoprim.

TECHNICAL NOTES

SYNERGISTIC NUTRIENTS

Vitamin B_3, betaine, choline, EPA, phosphatidyl-ethanolamine, folate, tryptophan.

INOSITOL HEXAPHOSPHATE

Most abundant inositol phosphate in plants.

Action: Chemopreventative and chemotherapeutic agent. Blocks epidermal growth factor induced by phosphatidyl inositol-3(P I-3) kinase activity.

STRUCTURE OF INOSITOL/ MYO-INOSITOL

cis-1,2,3,5-trans-4,6-Cyclohexanehexol
$C_6H_{12}O_6$

I	II	III
myo-Inositol	1L-*myo*-Inositol 1-phosphate	1D-*myo*-Inositol 1-phosphate

Isoflavones

(Diadzein, Genistein)

SOURCE
Soy beans, clover, alfalfa sprouts, chick peas, currants, flaxseeds, hazel nuts, passion fruit, peanuts, peas, prunes, raisins.

FUNCTIONS FACILITATED
Plays an important role in prevention of menopausal symptoms, osteoporosis, cancer and heart disease.

PROPOSED MECHANISM OF ACTION
Oestrogen modulator, induction of cancer cell differentiation, inhibitor of tyrosine kinase, inhibits lipoprotein oxidation, suppression of angiogenesis, antioxidant effects, inhibits nitric oxide synthetase, inhibits osteoclast acid secretion, inhibits angiogenesis and AP-1 transcription factor, up-regulates apoptotic signal Bax and down-regulates Bcl2, reverses arrest cycle progression at G2, inhibits topoisomerase II, a nuclear enzyme involved in DNA replication; inhibits glucose incorporation into nuclear ribose through non oxidative pentose cycle, reduces multi-drug resistance associated with chemotherapy.

Isoflavones protect tyrosine phosphatases, which alter the balance of protein phosphorylation – dephosphorylation reactions. Phosphorylation of protein by tyrosine kinases and other protein kinases escalates signal transduction pathways, which induce growth promotion, platelet aggregation, vascular smooth muscle hyperplasia and hypertrophy, resulting in increased vascular resistance and blood pressure.

Low dose (<50 mg/day)
Decreases cellular proliferation, increases endothelial NOS, increases vasodilation, increases osteoblastic activity, decreases endothelin 1, TGF beta activity, PSA and TNF response element; decreases progression of renal failure, protects against left ventricular hypertrophy, reduces risk of cancer (breast, prostate).

High dose (>80 mg/day)
Decreases lipid peroxidation and LDL cholesterol, induces uterine contractions, supports liver function.

THERAPEUTIC USES
Hot flushes, hypertension, menopausal symptoms, osteoporosis, prevention and treatment of breast, stomach, colon, and prostate cancer and leukaemia; reduces the risk of coronary artery disease.

DAILY DOSAGE	
SR	20-160 mg
Low dose	<50 mg/day Stimulates oestrogen receptor beta
High dose	>80 mg/day Stimulates oestrogen receptor alpha

DRUG/NUTRIENT INTERACTIONS
Isoflavones may alter the following drug activity:

Estrogen and estrogen-like medications – conjugated estrogens, estradiol, estrone, esterified estrogens, estropipate, ethinyl estradiol, raloxifene, transdermal estradiol, vaginal estrogens

Tamoxifen – soy isoflavone, genistein, may offset the ability of tamoxifen to inhibit estrogen responsive breast cancer tumor growth. Use with caution.

STRUCTURE OF ISOFLAVONES

4',5,7-Trihydroxyisoflavone; Genistein
$C_{15}H_{10}O_5$

Daidzein

Isoflavonoids are a group of diphenolic hormone-like compounds of dietary with anti-carcinogenic potency and anti coronary heart disease properties.

These isoflavonoids are derived mainly from soy-protein products, while clover seeds and leaves are a rich source of biochanin A and formononetin.

Genistein precursors, such as genistin and biochainin A, are converted by the intestinal microflora to genistein in the gut. Genistein is the aglycone (without sugar component) of the glycoside genistin.

The structure of genistein is similar to that of oestrogen. Genistein can act as a phyto-oestrogen, together with daidzein.

Lactobacillus

Acidophilus/Bifidobacterium

SOURCE

Fermented cabbage, yoghurt.

FACTORS INCREASING DEMAND

ADHD, antibiotics, atopic dermatitis, candida infections, constipation, chronic fatigue, irritable bowel syndrome, flatus, formula-fed infants, physical and emotional stress, thrush, radiation therapy of the bowel.

FUNCTIONS FACILITATED

Antimicrobial activity, anti-carcinogenic activity, antidiarrheal properties, decreases toxic bowel metabolites and improves liver detoxification, decreases oxidative stress, inhibits nitro-reductase, β-glucosidases and beta glucuronidase – the faecal bacterial enzyme responsible for deconjugating liver conjugated oestrogen; inactivates or inhibits carcinogenic compounds in the gut, improves immune competence, improves intestinal barrier defence, increases levels of circulating immunoglobulin A (IgA), lowers systemic inflammatory cytokines and potential neurotoxic compounds, production of short chain fatty acids for enterocyte energy, regulates bowel flora.

THERAPEUTIC USES

ADHD, antibiotic therapy, antibiotic associated diarrhoea, aphthous stomatitis, autism, breast cancer, candidiasis, chronic fatigue syndrome, cancer patients, colon cancer, constipation, diarrhoea, diverticular disease, elevated blood cholesterol, formula-fed infants, heart disease, infantile colic, inflammatory bowel disease, irritable bowel syndrome, recurrent vaginosis, stressed individuals, vomiting in children

Adjuvant treatment in major depressive disorders.

DRUG/NUTRIENT INTERACTIONS

Antibiotics – Aminoglycosides, Cephalosporins, Fluoroquinolones, Quinolones, Macrolides, Penicillins, Sulfonamides, Tetracyclines, Trimethoprin-containing antibiotics, Carbapenems, Monobactams, chloramphenicol, spectinomycin, Streptogramins, vancomycin, Oxalodinones, Lincosamides, Nitrofurans.

SYNERGISTIC NUTRIENTS

Fibre, fish oil (DHA/EPA), inulin, fructo-oligosaccharides, Lactobacillus casei, Lactobacillus plantarum, Lactobacillus rhamnosus, Bifidobacterium longum, Bifidobacteria breve, Streptococcus thermophilus.

Malic Acid

(Hydroxy succinic acid)

SOURCE
Apples, currants, most tart fruits.

DEFICIENCY MAY CAUSE OR BE ASSOCIATED WITH
Physical exhaustion, muscular pain, fibromyalgia.

FUNCTIONS FACILITATED
Activates pentose-phosphate cycle and tissue respiration enzymes, improves mitochondrial respiration, intermediate in the Krebs cycle, malate/aspartate shuttle.

THERAPEUTIC USES
Cisplatin induced nephrotoxicity, diabetes, endurance for athletic training, hepatotoxicity, musculoskeletal pain, fibromyalgia syndrome.

DAILY DOSAGE	
SR	300-1200 mg

SYNERGISTIC NUTRIENTS
Alpha ketoglutarate, biotin, magnesium, NAD.

DRUG/NUTRIENT INTERACTION
Cisplatin

STRUCTURE OF MALIC ACID

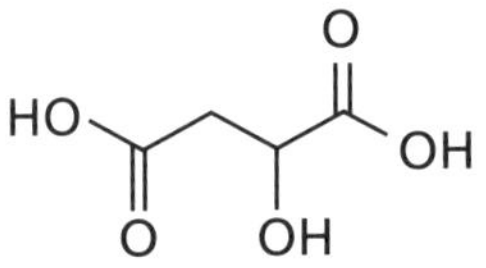

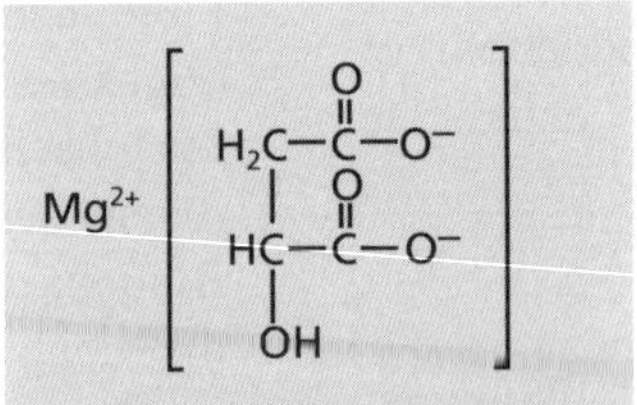

Magnesium Malate

Medium Chain Fatty Acids (MCFA)

SOURCE
Butter, coconut, palm oil.

FUNCTIONS FACILITATED
MCT = Median Chain triglycerides containing MCFA

Improves energy in patients with long-chain 3-hydroxyacyl-CoA dehydrogenase (LCHAD) and mitochondrial tri-functional protein (TFP) deficiency; provides an energy source that is rapidly oxidised; improves effectiveness of a ketogenic diet, protects EFAs and LC-PUFAs from ß-oxidation, improves energy intake in severely malnourished and malabsorbing patients after experiencing burns, trauma, surgery or severe infections; increases metabolic rate and thermogenesis, reduces weight gain in high fat diets, improves insulin sensitivity and glucose tolerance.

THERAPEUTIC USES
Biliary cirrhosis, cancer, cystic fibrosis, celiac disease, Crohn's disease, insulin resistance, ketogenic diets, obstructive jaundice, malabsorption in neonates, pancreatitis, metabolic syndrome, regional enteritis, weight loss, Whipple's disease.

Fatty acid Structures	
Fatty acid/Source	**Function**
SATURATED	
Butyric acid 4:0 Milk fat	Inhibits proliferation of colon cancer, induces differentiation of tumour cell; Inhibits histone deacetylase.
Caproic 6:0 Milk fat	**Medium Chain Fatty Acid (MCFA).** MCFAs and their derivatives act by disrupting the lipid membranes of the viruses; Reducing weight by reducing fat cell numbers; Helping conserve omega-3 fatty acid in tissues and normalizing the omega-6-to-omega-3 balance.
Caprylic Acid 8:0 Milk fat	MCFA
Capric acid 10:0 Milk fat, coconut	Medium Chain Fatty Acid (MCFA). Can be converted to monocaprin. Monocaprin has antiviral effects against HIV and is being tested for antiviral effects against herpes simplex and antibacterial effects against chlamydia and other sexually transmitted bacteria.

Fatty acid Structures

Fatty acid/Source	Function
Lauric acid 12:0 Coconut, palm kernel	Medium Chain Fatty Acid (MCFA). Lauric acid can be converted into monolaurin. Monolaurin is the antiviral, antibacterial, and antiprotozoal monoglyceride used by the human body to destroy lipid-coated viruses such as: HIV, herpes, cytomegalovirus, influenza, various pathogenic bacteria, including: listeria monocytogenes and helicobacter pylori, and protozoa such as: giardia lamblia; monolaurin induces proliferation of T cells and inhibits toxic shock syndrome toxin-1 mitogenic effects on T cells. Lauric acid has antimicrobial effects. "hypercholesterolemic saturated FA".
Myristic Acid 14:0 Milk fat, Coconut	Can raise total cholesterol and LDL-C plasma levels. "hypercholesterolemic saturated FA".
Palmitic acid 16:0 Plants and animals	Can raise total cholesterol and LDL-C plasma levels. "hypercholesterolemic saturated FA".
Stearic acid 18:0 Animal fat, cocoa butter	
MONO-UNSATURATED² **Palmitoleic acid** 16:1n-7 Most fats and oils	CH3(CH2)5CH=CH(CH2)7COOH
Oleic acid 18:1n-9 Most fats and oils, Almond oil, avocado, avocado oil, olive oil	Most common monounsaturated fatty acid in human cells, incorporated into cell membrane phospholipids, substrate for cellular energy production, enhances membrane fluidity compared to saturated fats, helps enhance hormone responsiveness, immuno-protective.

[1] Number of carbon (C) atoms: number of double bonds and position of the first double bond counting from the methyl (CH$_3$) end of the fatty acid

FATTY ACID STRUCTURES

Butyric Acid (C 4:0): $CH_3(CH_2)_2 COOH$

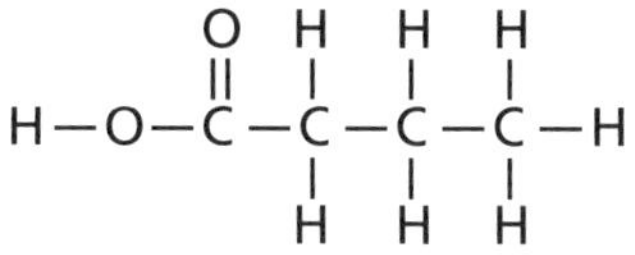

```
        O   H   H   H
        ||  |   |   |
H—O—C —C —C —C —H
        |   |   |
        H   H   H
```

Butyric acid-VFA

Caproic Acid (C 6:0): $CH_3(CH_2)_4 COOH$

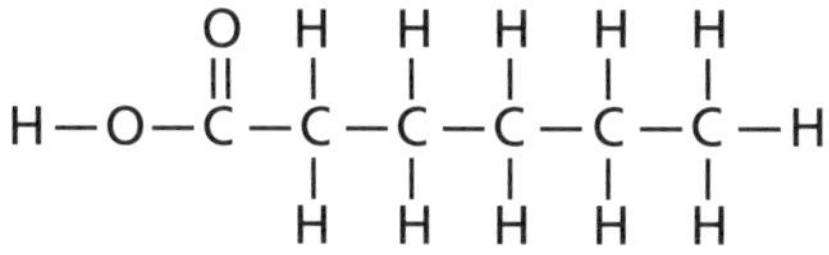

```
        O   H   H   H   H   H
        ||  |   |   |   |   |
H—O—C —C —C —C —C —C —H
        |   |   |   |   |
        H   H   H   H   H
```

Caproic Acid

Caprylic Acid (C 8:0): $CH_3(CH_2)_6 COOH$

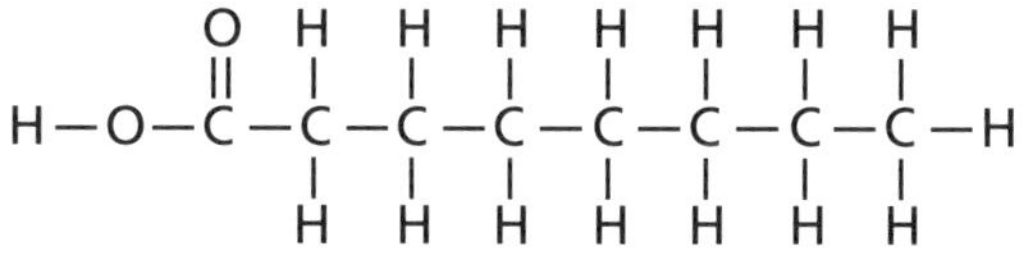

```
        O   H   H   H   H   H   H   H
        ||  |   |   |   |   |   |   |
H—O—C —C —C —C —C —C —C —C —H
        |   |   |   |   |   |   |
        H   H   H   H   H   H   H
```

Caprylic Acid

Capric Acid (C 10:0): $CH_3(CH_2)_8 COOH$

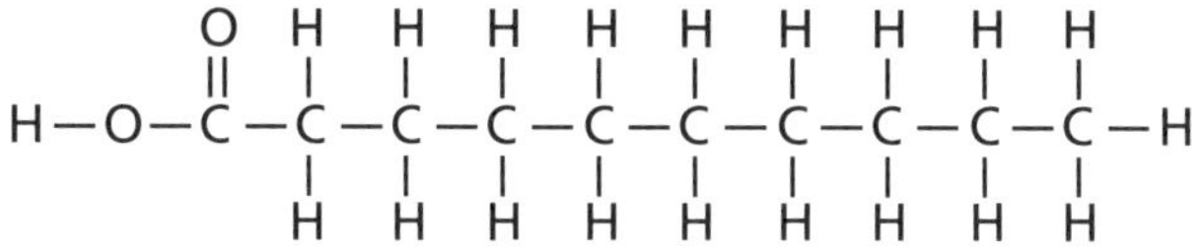

```
        O   H   H   H   H   H   H   H   H
        ||  |   |   |   |   |   |   |   |
H—O—C —C —C —C —C —C —C —C —C —C —H
        |   |   |   |   |   |   |   |   |
        H   H   H   H   H   H   H   H   H
```

Capric Acid

Lauric Acid (C 12:0): $CH_3(CH_2)_{10} COOH$

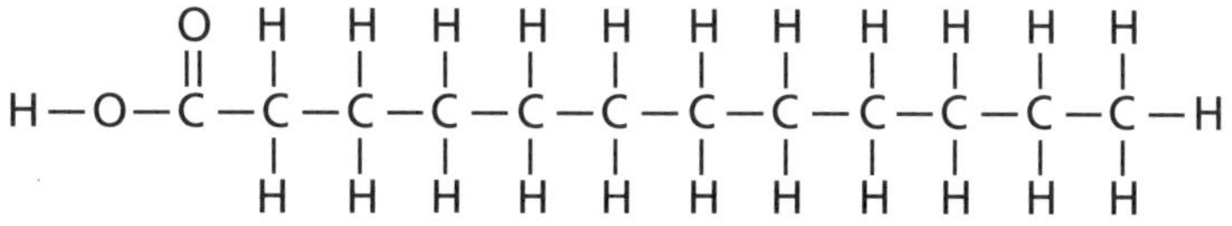

```
        O   H   H   H   H   H   H   H   H   H   H
        ||  |   |   |   |   |   |   |   |   |   |
H—O—C —C —C —C —C —C —C —C —C —C —C —C —H
        |   |   |   |   |   |   |   |   |   |   |
        H   H   H   H   H   H   H   H   H   H   H
```

Lauric Acid

Myristic Acid (C 14:0): $CH_3(CH_2)_{12}COOH$

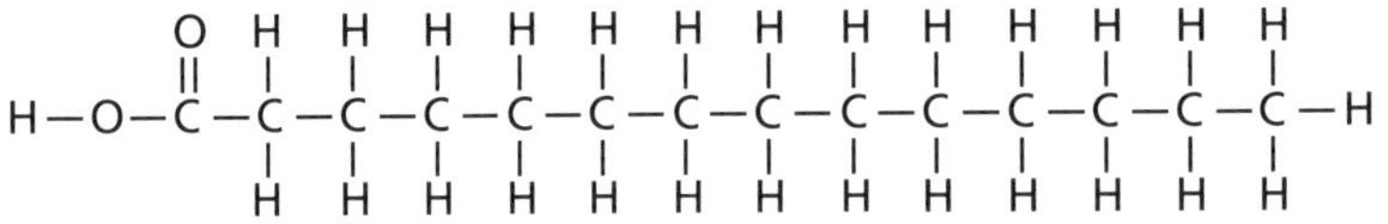

Myristic Acid

Palmitic Acid (C 16:0): $CH_3(CH_2)_{14}COOH$

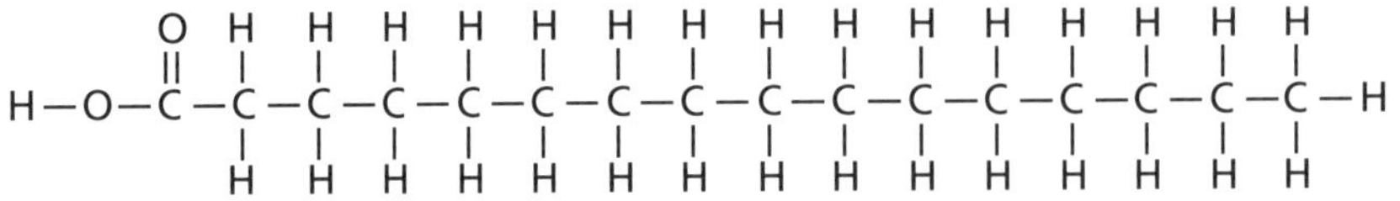

Palmitic Acid

Stearic Acid (C 18:0): $CH_3(CH_2)_{16}COOH$

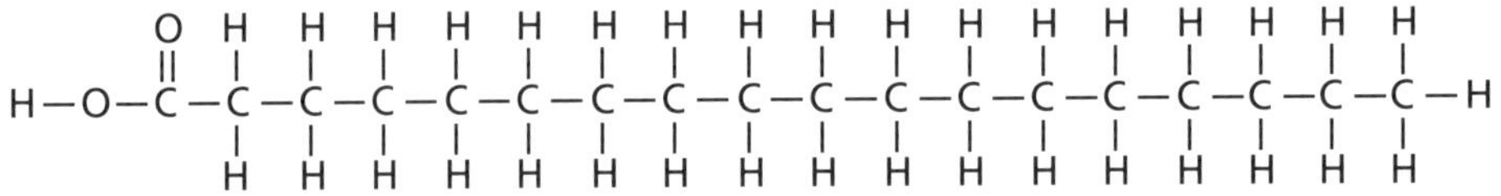

Stearic Acid

Oleic Acid (C 18:1): $CH_3(CH_2)_7CH=CH(CH_2)_7COOH$

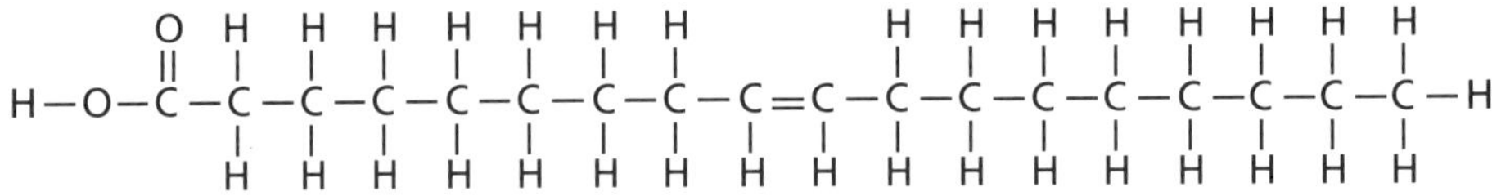

Oeic Acid-Monounsaturated Fatty Acid

Mucopoly-saccharides

(A source of chondroitin sulphate)

SOURCE
Aloe vera, cactus, calf tracheal cartilage, comfrey, ginseng, oatmeal, okra, pigs feet, raw oysters, shark cartilage, shellfish, slippery elm, tripe, wheat germ.

FUNCTIONS FACILITATED
Antibody synthesis, anti-anaphylactic effects, anti-tumour activity, growth stimulating effects, increases excretion of sodium, increases properdin levels, lipidaemia clearing effects, lubrication and cushioning of joints, maintains the strength and elasticity of arterial wells, provides a protective barrier in mucous membranes, wound healing and tissue regeneration, provides an aqueous matrix for diffusion of nutrients and electrolytes.

Muco-polysaccharides are found in all body tissues and fluids such as: blood group substances, blood vessels, cell walls, connective tissue, tendons, joints, intracellular ground substance and mucous membranes. Thus, its function is to provide structure and form.

COMPOSITION
Amino sugars.

There are over 100 different kinds of mucopolysaccharides.

Constituents include: Chondroitin sulfate A, B, and C, heparin, hyaluronic and keratan sulfate, sialic acid.

FACTORS INCREASING DEMAND
Age, arteriosclerosis, arthritis, coronary artery disease, defects in wound healing, infection, leprosy, rheumatoid arthritis, tuberculosis, scleroderma.

THERAPEUTIC USES
Acne, arthritis, asthma, back pain, bursitis, cancer, cartilage degeneration, Crohn's disease, colitis, diabetes, eczema, emphysema, hypertension, viral infections, warts, infertility, inflammatory conditions, poor bone healing, psoriasis, sunburn, ulcers, ulcerative colitis, wound healing.

DAILY DOSAGE	
SR	1500mg – 15g

DRUG/NUTRIENT INTERACTIONS
Cortisone, NSAIDs e.g. brufen, indomethacin.

N-acetyl-Cysteine (NAC)

SOURCE

Nutritional supplements.

FUNCTIONS FACILITATED

Acts as an antioxidant and scavenges hydrogen peroxide, hydroxy radical and hypochlorous acid; enhances T-cell function, heavy metal chelator, mucolytic, prevents metastasis by inhibiting gelatinase activity of type VI collagens, stimulates the synthesis of glutathione.

THERAPEUTIC USES

Acetaminophen (paracetamol) poisoning, ageing, AIDS, cancer therapy, chronic bronchitis, ethanol toxicity, heavy metal poisoning, hepatitis B, infertility, lung fibrosis, metastasis, motor neuron disease, Sjogren's syndrome, smokers, viral myocarditis.

DAILY DOSAGE

SR	100-1500mg

DRUG/ NUTRIENT INTERACTIONS

Doxorubicin, oxazaphosphorines, nataminophen, zidovudine, bleomycin, adriamycin, cyclophosphamide, ifosfamide, nitroglycerin

SYNERGISTIC NUTRIENTS

Zinc, cysteine, glutathione.

STRUCTURE OF N-ACETYL CYSTEINE

N-acetylcysteine (NAC) is a thiol, in which the hydrogen atom can act to reduce free radicals.

Ornithine

Non essential amino acid, breakdown product of arginine

FUNCTIONS FACILITATED

Detoxifies ammonia, increases insulin and growth hormone levels, increases the efficiency of energy consumption and promotes the excretion of ammonia, promotes tissue repair, precursor to poly amines, reduces body fat, required for the synthesis of citrulline, proline and glutamic acid.

THERAPUTIC USES

Activates urea cycle, ageing (combats muscle loss with age), anti-fatigue factor, body builders, cirrhosis, intense physical exercise, physical fatigue, promotes lipid metabolism, surgery, trauma.

DAILY DOSAGE	
SR	1-5 g/day

SYNERGISTIC NUTRIENTS

Arginine, carnitine, alpha keto gluterate

Orotic Acids and Salts

SOURCE
Human breast milk, milk, whey.

FUNCTIONS FACILITATED
Actively involved in mineral transport, involved in the synthesis of ribonucleotides (RNA, DNA), promotes growth, stimulates the rate of certain metabolic pathways - increases the concentration of various pyrimidine cofactors involved in lipid and carbohydrate metabolism.

THERAPEUTIC USES	
Calcium orotate	Arteriosclerosis, arthritis, disseminated encephalitis, fractures, hypertension, osteoporosis, phlebitis, regulation of blood calcium levels, retinitis, spondylarthritis. Calcium orotate seems to have significant anti-inflammatory effects.
Magnesium orotate	Arteriosclerosis, arrhythmias, heart failure, hypertension, lipidaemia.
Orotic Acid	Hyperlipidaemia, myocardial infarction, neonatal jaundice, pernicious anaemia, surgery and wound healing.
Potassium orotate	Angina, chronic cardiovascular disease, heart failure, high blood cholesterol, hypertension.

DAILY DOSAGE	
SR	300-1000 mg

STRUCTURE OF OROTIC ACID

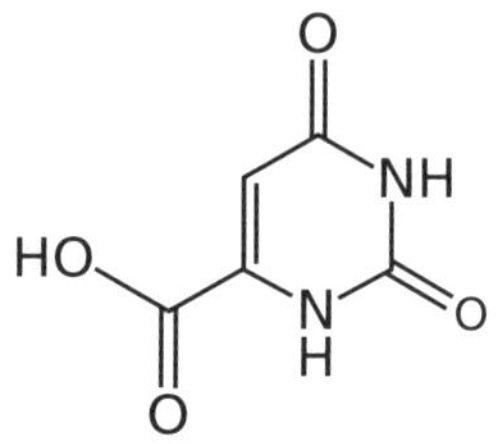

Pyrimidine carboxylic acid,
S-Dihydroorotate;
(S)-4,5-Dihydroorotate;
L-Dihydroorotate;
L-Dihydroorotic acid;
Dihydro-L-orotic acid

Pyrimidinecarboxylic acid, also known as **orotic acid** or vitamin B13. Historically it was believed to be a vitamin but this is now known not to be the case. It is manufactured in the body by intestinal flora. It is a good carrier for minerals such as: lithium, magnesium, calcium and potassium and makes them more bioavailable for cellular uptake.

Pancreatic Enzymes

SOURCE

Pancreas or its juices, pancreatin tablets.

FUNCTION OF VARIOUS ENZYMATIC CONSTUENTS	
Carboxypeptidase A and B	Both activated by trypsin; these enzymes cleave carboxy terminal amino acids with aromatic, branched aliphatic and basic side chains respectively from proteins and polypeptides.
Chymotrypsin	Activated by trypsin; chymotrypsin cleaves peptide bonds adjacent to aromatic, hydrophobic amino acids of proteins and polypeptides.
Elastase	Activated by trypsin; elastase cleaves those bonds of elastin and some other proteins that are adjacent to alanine, glycine, and serine.
Pancreatic alpha-	Activated by chloride ions (from amylasestomach HCl secretion); this enzyme hydrolyses 1, 4 -alpha linkages of starches.
Pancreatic Lipase	Activated by emulsifying agents; this lipase breaks down triglycerides (fats) to form mono and diglycerides.
Phospholipase	Activated by trypsin; this enzyme produces lysolecithin from lecithin.
Ribonuclease and Deoxyribonuclease	These enzymes cleave the bonds of RNA and DNA respectively to form nucleotides.
Trypsin	Activated by enterokinase; trypsin cleaves peptide bonds adjacent to arginine and lysine in proteins and polypeptides.

FACTORS INCREASING DEMAND

Allergy, cancer, cystic fibrosis, excess flatus, food intolerances, inflammation, intestinal surgery, liver disorders, malnutrition, marasmus, pancreatitis, shift workers, steatorrhoea, stress.

THERAPEUTIC USES

Anorexia, arthritis, asthma, cancer, cystic fibrosis, diabetes, diarrhoea, Down's syndrome, eczema and related skin disorders, food intolerances, intestinal surgery, intestinal wind, liver and pancreatic disorders, multiple sclerosis, protein calorie malnutrition.

NOTE: Functions best in alkaline conditions. Bicarbonate one hour after meals may improve function of these enzymes.

Para-amino-benzoic Acid

(PABA)

SOURCE

Brewer's yeast, brown rice, eggs, fish, kidney, liver, wholegrain cereals, wheat germ, sunflower seeds, yoghurt.

FACTORS INCREASING DEMAND

Excessive sun exposure, phototoxicity, ozone pollution exposure, rickettsial diseases.

FUNCTIONS FACILITATED

Constituent of folic acid, enhances antitumour activity of ionizing radiation, intestinal bacterial activity, restores greying hair, aids in the assimilation of pantothenic acid.

DEFICIENCY MAY CAUSE OR BE ASSOCIATED WITH:

Constipation, depression, digestive disorders, fatigue, greying hair, irritability.

THERAPEUTIC USES

Applied topically acts as a sun block; chemically sensitive individuals, detoxifies hydroquinone and phenyl-arsenates, eczema, greying hair, ozone exposure, photosensitivity, radiation therapy, rickets.

DAILY DOSAGE	
RDA	None given
SR	10-1000 mg

EFFECTS OF OVERDOSAGE AND TOXICITY
Sensitivity in some individuals – check liver function.
Anorexia, fever, nausea, skin rash.

TECHNICAL NOTES

SYNERGISTIC NUTRIENTS

Vitamin B_5, folic acid.

DRUG/NUTRIENT INTERACTIONS
Alcohol, Antibiotics – sulphonamides, hydroquinone, phenyl arsenate.

STRUCTURE OF PARA AMINO BENZOIC ACID (PABA)

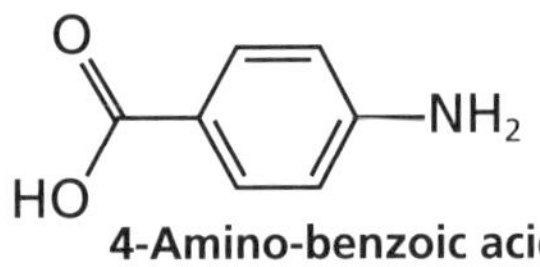

4-Amino-benzoic acid

p-Aminobenzoic acid is a part of folic acid molecule. It was called Vitamin BX as it is a component of pteroylglutamate. However, it does not contribute to synthesize folate in human body.

Pepsin

SOURCE

The stomach.

Formulated digestive aids generally contain betaine, glutamic acid, HCI and pepsin.

FUNCTION

Activated by hydrochloric acid (HCI), pepsin cleaves peptide bonds of proteins and polypeptides that are adjacent to aromatic amino acids; reduces transforming growth factor beta.

FACTORS INCREASING DEMAND

Achlorhydria, ageing, alcohol, antacid abuse, cancer, indigestion.

THERAPEUTIC USES

Alcoholics, achlorhydria, ageing, candidiasis, cancer patients, epigastric fullness, food intolerances, gastric mucosal atrophy, gastric surgery, hiatus hernia, indigestion, gas and belching, multiple myeloma.

NOTE: Works best in acid environment.

SYNERGISTIC NUTRIENTS

Iron.

Phosphatidyl Serine

Contingent nutrient

SOURCE
Soy lecithin, egg lecithin.

FACTORS INCREASING DEMAND
De-myelinating diseases, multiple sclerosis, viral or bacterial encephalitis.

FUNCTIONS FACILITATED
Decreases cortisol excretion during intense exercise, facilitates nerve cell function, improves memory, learning and concentration; improves the release of dopamine, noradrenaline and acetylcholine, improves exercise capacity, inhibits tumour necrosing factor, maintains flexibility of cell membranes, neurotransmitter release and synaptic activity, normalises age related neurotransmitter receptor abnormalities, stimulates the synthesis of nerve growth factor.

THERAPEUTIC USES
Ageing, Alzheimer's disease, athletic performance, autoimmune demyelinating diseases, CNS inflammation, cognitive failure, dementia, encephalitis (viral, bacterial), intense stressful exercise, multiple sclerosis, Parkinson's disease, poor memory.

DAILY DOSAGE	
SR	100-800 mg/day

SYNERGISTIC NUTRIENTS
Vitamin B_{12}, folic acid.

STRUCTURE OF PHOSPHATIDYL SERINE

Phosphatidylserine;
Phosphatidyl-I -serine;
1,2-Diacyl-sn-glycerol - 3-phospho - L - serine;
3-O-sn-Phosphatidyl-L-serine;
O3-Phosphatidyl-L-serine

Pyrroloquinoline Quinone (PQQ)

(Methoxatin) Contingent nutrient

SOURCE
Cocoa powder, colostrum, broad beans, green pepper, Kiwi fruit, pawpaw, parsley, tofu, tea, spinach.

FACTORS INCREASING DEMAND
Excessive chick pea intake, pregnancy, neonates.

FUNCTIONS FACILITATED
Acts as an antioxidant, protects against oxidative stress, scavenges superoxide and peroxide, increases glutathione (GSH) in liver and eye lens, inhibits tyrosine transcription by MSH (melanocyte stimulating hormone), co-factor for the enzyme lysyl oxidase which is involved in the cross linking of collagen and elastin, maintains skin integrity, co-factor in the NADH- ubiquinone reductase system in the mitochondria, stimulates nerve growth factor, involved in the respiratory bursts of neutrophils, which destroys bacteria and helps maintain normal immune function; protects neurones from NMDA receptor-mediated glutamate excitotoxicity, protects magno-cellular cholinergic neurons (involved in memory and learning) in the basal forebrain, can substitute for vitamin B2 in some reactions, stimulates mitochondrial Complex 1 activity, reduces brain hypoxia in stroke, improves T and B cell mitogen response, reduces iNOS expression.

TARGET TISSUES
Neutrophils, monocytes, CSF, heart, lens and eye tissue, liver.

DEFICIENCY SYMPTOMS
Abdominal haemorrhages, aortic aneurisms, friable skin, hair loss, reduced levels of lysyl oxidase activity, decreased immunity, decreases size and number of mitochondria, diverticula, hunched posture, increase in blood sugar, sterility, weight loss.

THERAPEUTIC USES
Alzheimer's disease, chemical exposure, chemical liver damage, dementia, poor immunity, poor memory and learning, exposure to carbon tetrachloride, poor skin integrity, aneurism, stroke, ischaemic brain damage.

DAILY DOSAGE	
SR	100-400 ug

Note: High dose can initiate increase in free radical production resulting in DNA damage.

EFFECTS OF OVER DOSAGE OR TOXICITY
Nephrotoxicity, oxidative damage

SYNERGISTIC NUTRIENTS
Vitamin B_2, B_3, Co enzyme Q_{10}, glycine, tryptophan, tyrosine, glutamine, vitamin C, glutathione, copper.

ENZYMES SYSTEMS INVOLVED
- Glucose dehydrogenase – oxidises glucose to gluconolactone.
- Methanol dehydrogenase.
- Lysyl oxidase.

STRUCTURE OF PYRROLOQUINOLINE QUINONE

Pyrroloquinoline quinone (PQQ) is a tricyclic o-quinone.

PQQ is highly soluble, heat-stable and capable of continuous redox cycling. The chemical properties of PQQ are analogous to combining some of the best chemical features of ascorbic acid (reducing potential), riboflavin (redox reactions), and pyridoxal (PL) (carbonyl reactivity) cofactors into one molecule.

R-Lipoic Acid

Contingent nutrient

SOURCE

Broccoli, kidney, garden peas, heart, liver, potatoes, rice bran, spinach, tomatoes.

FACTORS INCREASING DEMAND

Amanita mushroom poisoning, diabetes, doxorubicin, emphysema, heart disease, HIV infection, liver disease.

FUNCTIONS FACILITATED

Metabolic antioxidant, helps recycle antioxidants, vitamin C, E, CoQ_{10} and glutathione, improves ATP synthesis, increases T lymphocyte production, increases T helper: T suppressor ratio, inhibits the production of nuclear factor Kappa-B, quenches peroxynitrite, hydroxyl, singlet oxygen and HOCl radicals; reduces insulin resistance and improves glucose metabolism, reduces neural damage associated with excitatory amino acid toxicity and diabetes, supports mitochondrial function, detoxifies the body of heavy metal pollutants e.g. cadmium, lead, mercury; acts as a water and fat-soluble antioxidant, reduces glycation reactions, reverses the declines in oxygen consumption and mitochondrial energy production associated with ageing, co-factor for mitochondrial dehydrogenase, neuro-protective agent, elevates intracellular glutathione levels, regulates neuronal calcium homeostasis, regulates pro-inflammatory cytokines, decreases ICAM and VCAM expression, recruits glucose transporter 4 on cell membranes, co-factor for mitochondrial enzymes – catalyses oxidative decarboxylation of pyruvate, alpha ketoglutarate, alpha keto acids and branch chain amino acids; inhibits advanced glycation end products, inhibits pyruvate dehydrogenase kinase (PDK1>PDK4>PDK2>PDK3) – this inhibition stimulates mitochondrial burning of glucose and reduction in lactate production; may improve mitochondrial metabolism in cancer cells thus reducing proliferation, improves intercellular vitamin C levels, prevents pancreatic Beta cell destruction associated with diabetes type 1, insulin sensitizer.

THERAPEUTIC USES

AIDS, ageing, aged related memory deficits, Alzheimer's disease, amanita mushroom poisoning, asthma, atherosclerosis, cataracts, cancer cachexia, chronic fatigue, cognitive decline, dementia, diabetic cardiomyopathy, diabetes, diabetic neuropathy, emphysema, ischaemic heart disease, Huntington's disease, inflammation, insulin resistance, kidney damage, loss of smell, multiple sclerosis, neurodegeneration, nerve damage, open angle glaucoma, Parkinson's disease, peripheral neuropathy, poor memory, rheumatoid arthritis, radiation injury, radiation sickness, sports nutrition, stroke, vision problems, weight control, disease complications of diabetes e.g. heart disease.

DAILY DOSAGE	
SR	100-600mg for diabetics
	20-50mg for anti-oxident effect

Note 1: Take 60 minutes before meals or 2 hours after meals. High doses of lipoic acid may compete with biotin in some reactions. Biotin supplementation is warranted with high dose lipoic acid supplementation.

Note 2: Lipoic acid has a 1/2 life of 30 minutes in the blood.

SYNERGISTIC NUTRIENTS

CoQ_{10}, vitamins E, C, glutathione, NAD, N-acetyl cysteine, biotin, acetyl-l-carnitine.

Side effects of high dose include: nausea, fatigue & insomnia, mal-odorous urine produced from octanoic acid & cysteine.

STRUCTURE OF LIPOIC ACID

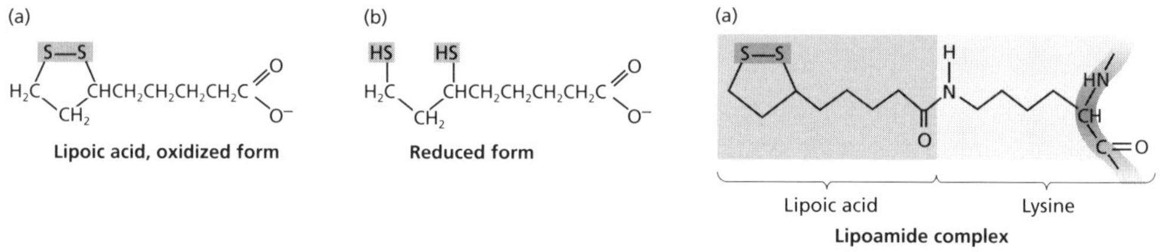

(a)

Lipoic acid, oxidized form

(b)

Reduced form

(a)

Lipoic acid   Lysine

Lipoamide complex

Lipoic acid exists as a mixture of two structures: a closed-ring disulfide form and an open-chain reduced form. Oxidation-reduction cycles interconvert these two species. As is the case for biotin, lipoic acid does not often occur free in nature, but rather is covalently attached in amide linkage with lysine residues on enzymes. The enzyme that catalyses the formation of the *lipoamide* linkage, requires ATP and produces lipoamide-enzyme conjugates, AMP, and pyrophosphate as products of the reaction.

Lipoic acid is an acyl group carrier. It is found in pyruvate dehydrogenase and alpha-ketoglutarate dehydrogenase, two multienzyme complexes involved in carbohydrate metabolism.

Lipoic acid functions to couple acyl-group transfer and electron transfer during oxidation and decarboxylation of alpha-keto acids.

R and S Form of Lipoic Acid

Unlike the natural form, the S-lipoic acid does not improve cellular ATP levels. The R-form increases membrane fluidity while the S-form decreases fluidity.

The S form potentiates the deterioration of the lens in diabetes.

Resveratrol

(3,4',5-trihydroxystilbene)

SOURCE

Grapes, red wine, grape juice, peanuts, and berries of *Vaccinum* species, including blueberries, bilberries, and cranberries; rhubarb, white hellebore (Veratrium grandiflorum)

FUNCTIONS FACILITATED

Acts as antioxidant, anti-inflammatory, blocks the multistep process of carcinogenesis; reduces coronary artery disease, inhibits LDL oxidation; inhibits the expression of adhesion molecules; inhibits platelet aggregation; inhibits certain cytochrome P450 enzymes, increases phase 2 detox pathway (increases expression and activity of NADPH:quinine oxidase); induces cell cycle arrest and induces apoptosis in some cancer cell lines (breast, prostate, stomach, colon, pancreatic and thyroid cancers); lowers the levels of secreted and intracellular amyloid- (A) peptides; modulates cyclooxygenase and lipoxygenase activity; possess estrogenic activity (acts as a phytoestrogen); stimulate eNOS activity in cultured endothelial cells; suppresses PSA; upregulates p53 and Bax; suppresses NF-KB, AP-1, inhibits protein kinases. Inhibits voltage gated sodium channels and increases mitogenesis; chemo-preventative (anti-cancer agent), anti-ageing effects, prevents cell proliferation, cardio-protective, suppresses ROS production in endothelial cells, activates SIRT-1.

THERAPEUTIC USES

Aging, Alzheimer's disease; atherosclerosis, cardiac hypertrophy, enhances the anti-tumour effects of gemcitabine, high-fat diets, nephrotic syndrome; prevention of the following cancers: (colon, liver, osteo sarcoma, pancreas, prostate, stomach and thyroid), melanoma, metabolic syndrome, myeloid leukemic cells, head and neck squamous cell carcinomas, ovarian carcinoma and cervical carcinoma; augments the apoptotic activity of chemotherapeutic agents and radiation.

DAILY DOSAGE	
SR	200-1400mg/day

TARGET ORGANS

Liver and Kidney

SYNERGISTIC NUTRIENTS

Quercetin

Supplementation Range- 100mg/kg of body weight

STRUCTURE OF RESVERATROL
(3,4',5- TRIHYDROXYSTILBENE)

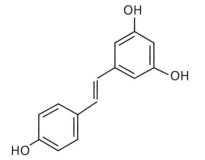

Molecular Formula: $C_{14}H_{12}O_3$
Molecular Weight: 228.247
Appearance: White solid
Melting Point: 253-255°C
Solubility: Readily soluble in water
Chemical Name: trans-3,4',5-trihydroxystilbene

International non-proprietary name: Resveratrol

S-adenosyl-methionine (SAMe)

Contingent nutrient

SOURCE
Supplements

FACTORS INCREASING DEMAND
Endogenous depression, liver disease.

Intake of the following drugs: L-dopa, acetaminophen, oestrogen, calcium, channel blockers, cardizem, diltiazem.

FUNCTIONS FACILITATED
Converts noradrenaline to adrenaline, involved in the synthesis of creatine, Co enzyme Q_{10}, carnitine, glutathione, polyamines, heat shock proteins and cytokines; methylates DNA, converts phosphatidyl ethanolamine to phosphatidyl choline, protects and enhances cell integrity, regulates cell growth.

S-adenosyl methionine is formed from the amino acid methionine and acts as a major methyl donor in many biochemical methylation reactions as part of hepatic phase II detoxification.

THERAPEUTIC USES
Ageing, alcohol toxicity, anxiety, arthritic pain, biliary obstruction, cirrhosis, cholestasis depression, Down's syndrome, fatty liver, fibromyalgia, hepatitis, liver cancer, Parkinson's disease.

DAILY DOSAGE

SR	200-1000 mg/day

Note: Some bipolar patients act adversely to SAMe supplementation, thus it should be given under doctor's supervision.

SYNERGISTIC NUTRIENTS
Betaine, folic acid, vitamin B_6.

DRUG/NUTRIENT INTERACTIONS

SAMe may reduce the dosage of anti-depressants –fluoxetine, fluvoxamine, paroxetine, sertraline, amitriptyline, amoxapine, clomipramine, desipramine, doxepin, imipramine, nortriptyline, trimipramine, maprotiline, mirtazapine, trazodone, bupropion, venlafaxine, nefazodone, citalopram, protriptyline, phenelzine, tranylcypromine, isocarboxazid.

Use with caution if taken together.

Decreases SAMe in the CNS:
   Levodopa

STRUCTURE OF S-ADENOSYL METHIONINE

S-Adenosylmethionine $C_{15}H_{22}N_6O_5S$

S-adenosyl-L-methionine (SAMe) is a natural substance present in the cells of the body. It is a direct metabolite of the essential amino acid L-methionine. It is variously known as ademetionine, S-adenosylmethione, SAM, SAMe and SAM-e.

SAME is highly unstable at temperatures above 0 degree C. Since the 1970s, certain salts of SAMe have become available that are stable at higher temperatures. These forms, which are clearly more desirable, include SAMe para-toluene sulphonates and SAMe 1,4 butanedisulfonate. These more stable forms have been used in many of the SAMe studies. However, even these temperature-stable forms must be kept very dry since moisture can cause hydrolysis. Stable, enteric-coated tablets are recommended.

Salicylic acid/ Acetyl-salicylic Acid

SOURCE

Organic vegetables and fruits, spices, herbs, European Juneberries.

FUNCTIONS FACILITATED

Anti inflammatory action, anti neoplastic actions, co-ordinately inhibits the activity of NF-αB, activates heat shock transcription factor 1 and suppresses cytokine gene expression in activated monocytes and macrophages, down-regulates the production of fibrinogen, fibronectin, and α–hemolysin — virulence factors necessary for bacterial replication in host tissues; inhibits the expression of genes for TNFα, IL-1ß, IL-6, IL-8, IL-10, and ICAM-1 in monocytes activated by the proinflammatory LPS; inhibits cyclooxygenase-1 (COX-1) activity, thereby the synthesis of pro-inflammatory and potentially-neoplastic prostaglandins (PGE2); reduces platelet aggregation.

FACTORS INCREASING DEMAND

Aging, atherosclerosis, arthritis, cardiovascular disease, colon cancer, type-2 diabetes.

THERAPEUTIC USES

Alzheimer's disease, cardiovascular disease, chemoprevention of colon cancer, giant cell arteritis, thrombosis, lipid induced insulin resistance, secondary prevention of cerebrovascular incidents, endovascular infections, headaches, pre-eclampsia.

DAILY DOSAGE	
Dietary Intake	10-100 mg/day
SR	100-3000mg/day

High dosage > 150 mg can increase side effects.

SIDE EFFECTS

Haemorrhagic episodes, gastrointestinal irritation and bleeding, increases bleeding time, inhibits the liver enzyme phenol sulfotransferases.

There is a suggestion that salicylic acid or aspirin should not be taken by children with fever as it may induce Reye's syndrome.

SYNERGISTIC NUTRIENTS

Calcium, magnesium and glycine reduce the side effects of salicylates.

Folic acid, DHA/EPA.

DRUG/NUTRIENT INTERACTIONS
Alcohol, methotrexate, wafarin

Tetrahydro-biopterin (Bh4)

Contingent nutrient

SOURCE

Meats

FACTORS INCREASING DEMAND

Phenylketonuria (certain variants only).

FUNCTIONS FACILITATED

Co-factor for – phenylalanine hydroxylase, tyrosine hydroxylase, tryptophan hydroxylase, nitric oxide synthase and alkyl glycerol mono-oxygenase; involved in the synthesis of neurotransmitters – serotonin, dopamine and noradrenaline; involved in apoptosis and other cellular events mediated by nitric oxide production, plays a role in proliferation and differentiation of erythroid cells, acts as a neurotransmitter-releasing factor for dopamine and acetylcholine, protects dopaminergic neurons from oxidative stress.

DEFICIENCY MAY CAUSE OR BE ASSOCIATED WITH:

Diabetes, decreased nitric oxide synthesis resulting in endothelial dysfunction, phenylketonuria, vascular injury.

THERAPEUTIC USES

Anxiety, Alzheimer's disease, cognitive dysfunction, depression, dementia, dopamine responsive dystonia, diabetes, insulin resistance, hyperlipidaemia, hypertension, schizophrenia phenylketonuria.

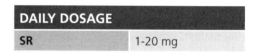

DAILY DOSAGE	
SR	1-20 mg

Note: High dose folic acid may be able to replace Bh_4 in some reactions.

SYNERGISTIC NUTRIENTS

Folic acid, B_{12}, B_6, magnesium, sepiapterin, 5-methyl-tetrahydrofolate.

TARGET TISSUES

Blood, spleen, lung, brain.

STRUCTURE OF TERAHYDROBIOPTERIN

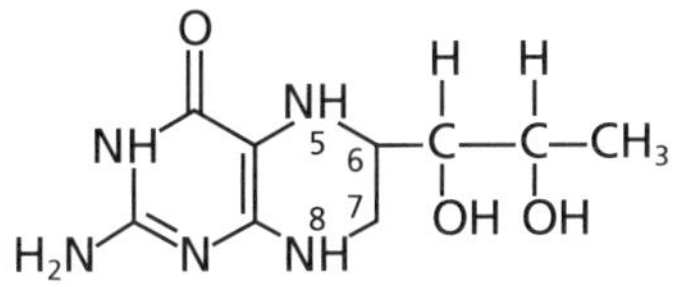

5,6,7-Tetrahydrobiopterin

Dihydrobiopterin

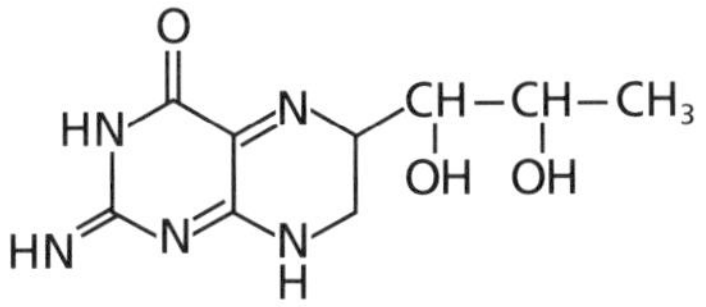

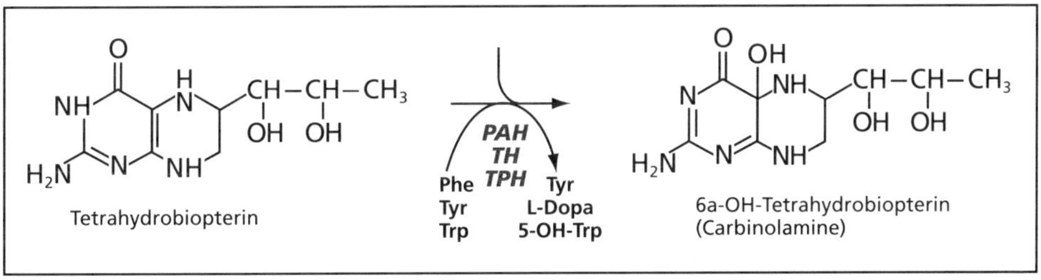

Tetrahydrobiopterin

PAH
TH
TPH

Phe → Tyr
Tyr → L-Dopa
Trp → 5-OH-Trp

6a-OH-Tetrahydrobiopterin
(Carbinolamine)

The structure of 5-methyltetrahydrofolate is similar to tetrahydrobiopterin and both agents have been shown to improve endothelium-dependent vasodilatation.

Xylitol

SOURCE

Raspberries, strawberries, chicory, cauliflower, lettuce.

FUNCTIONS FACILITATED

Inhibits the growth of detrimental organisms, helps to maintain bone density, retards demineralisation of tooth enamel, suppresses growth of detrimental bacteria, which cause tooth decay, facilitates intestinal absorption of calcium, used as a sweetener – does not increase blood glucose levels, suppresses helicobacter pylori, enhances thermogenesis.

THERAPEUTIC USES

Otitis media, osteoporosis, dry mouth, tooth decay, diabetes, helicobacter pylori, obesity.

DAILY DOSAGE	
SR	up to 40g per day

STRUCTURE OF XYLITOL

CHAPTER 5

Toxic Metals

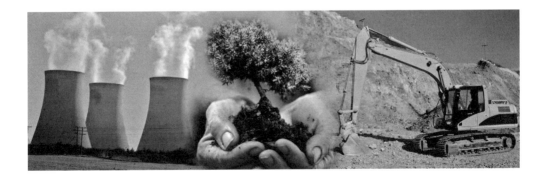

Aluminium (Al)

SOURCE

Aluminium cans, antacids, anti-diarrhoea medications, antiperspirants, baking powder, buffered analgesics, aluminium cooking vessels, cigarette filters, fabric softeners, food additives, nasal sprays, softened water, tea, table salt, toothpaste, vaccinations, vaginal douches.

Aluminium silicate clays - montmorillonite, bentonite, kaolinite and erionite.

SUSCEPTIBILITY INCREASED IN:

Babies, children, chronic renal insufficiency, low birth-weight infants, phosphate deficiency, zinc deficiency, iron deficiency.

Citric acid increases aluminium absorption.

Approximately 9% of the population have high body burden of aluminium.

ANTAGONISTS

Vitamins C, D, calcium, iron, magnesium, malic acid, phosphorus, selenium, zinc.

MECHANISM OF TOXICITY

Aluminium is capable of producing a biphasic effect on diverse cell systems. High doses inhibit and low doses stimulate various enzyme systems.

Aluminium induces mitochondrial dysfunction particularly in Hepatocytes; increases the expression of lipogenic enzymes; activates hypoxic inducing factor; activates anaerobic glycolysis.

Aluminium activates HIF1 and activates anabolic glycolysis.

Aluminium induces mitochondrial dysfunction.

Induces microcytic anaemia, inhibits hexokinase, inhibits phosphorus absorption, interferes with the slow axonal transmission of neurofilaments, reduces total bone and matrix formation, aluminium interacts with calcium in bone and kidneys, resulting in aluminium osteodystrophy; accumulates in neuronal plaques, inhibitor of cholinesterase (biphasic effect), interferes with choline transport (this may lead to acetylcholine deficiency), behavioural toxin, promotes formation and accumulation of insoluble A beta and hyper-phosphorylated taurine, mimics the deficit of cortical cholinergic neurotransmission seen in Alzheimer's disease, increases Fe-induced oxidative injury, interacts with calcium in bone and kidneys, resulting in aluminium osteodystrophy.

Calcium deficiency along with low dietary magnesium may contribute to aluminium-induced degenerative nervous disease.

No known physiologic need exists for aluminium; however, because of its atomic size and electric charge (0.051 nm and 3+, respectively), it is sometimes a competitive inhibitor of several essential elements of similar characteristics, such as magnesium (0.066 nm, 2+), calcium (0.099 nm, 2+), and iron (0.064 nm, 3+). Approximately 95% of an aluminium load becomes bound to transferrin and albumin intravascularly and is then eliminated via the kidneys.

SYMPTOMS OF TOXICITY

Alzheimer's disease, amyotrophic lateral sclerosis (ALS), anorexia, ataxia, bone fractures, bone pain, colic, decreases bone density, cognitive decline, dyslexia, dementia, gastroenteritis, hypophosphataemia, increases calcium dementia, increases calcium excretion, liver dysfunction, muscle pain, microcytic hypochromic anaemia, nephritis, neurodegenerative disease, osteodystrophy, osteomalacia, osteoporosis, Parkinson's disease, psychosis, rickets, resistance to vitamin D therapy, senile dementia, seizures, weakness, dialysis encephalopathy (a progressive form of dementia characterized by tremors, convulsions, psychosis and other changes in speech and behaviour – associated with long-term haemodialysis).

DAILY EXPOSURE

20-100 mg/day

Note: The aluminium concentration in muscle, bone and brain of patients maintained on a phosphorus binding Al gel for at least two years was respectively 14.8, 95.5 and 6.5 µg/g dry-weight. In control subjects levels were 1.2, 2.4 and 2.2 µg/g dry-weight.

Patients on dialysis, who died of a neurologic syndrome of unknown cause (dialysis encephalopathy syndrome), had brain grey matter concentrations of 25 mg Al/kg dry weight, while in controls 2.2 mg/kg was measured.

DOSAGE OF AL THAT INCREASES RISK OF TOXICITY

1.5-3.4gm/day

ABSORPTION

Oral aluminium bioavailability from water appears to be about 0.3%, from oral intake of food approximately 2%.

Aluminium is absorbed from the GI tract in the form of oral phosphate-binding agents (aluminium hydroxide), parenterally via immunizations, via dialysate or total parenteral nutrition (TPN) contamination, via the urinary mucosa through bladder irrigation, and transdermally in antiperspirants.

Lactate, citrate, and ascorbate all facilitate GI absorption. If a significant load exceeds the body's excretory capacity, the excess is deposited in various tissues, including: bone, brain, liver, heart, spleen, and muscle. This accumulation causes morbidity and mortality through various mechanisms.

Note: Calcium deficiency along with low dietary magnesium may contribute to aluminium-induced neuron disease.

EXCRETION

Renal excretion is increased by citric acid, malic acid (malate), and succinic acid (succinate), but they also increase aluminium absorption.

Most aluminium is excreted through the bowel.

MEDICAL TREATMENT

Deferoxamine mesylate or calcium disodium edetate (EDTA) chelation.

Arsenic (As)

*Arsenic at very low doses acts as a nutrient.

SOURCE

Cereals and breads, clams, drinking water, fish, meat, oysters, chinese and ayurvedic herbs, sea food.

Organic arsenic, also known as fish or seaweed arsenic (arsenocholine, arsenobetaine, or arsenosugars), is mostly found in seafood such as bivalves, bottom-feeding fish, and seaweed and has a lower toxicity.

Medical forms of arsenic: arsenic trioxide (As_2O_3).

Environmental sources: pesticides, fuel oils, weed killers, copper smelting, wood preservative, manufacture of glass and ceramics.

Permissible Exposure Limit = 10 µg/m³ (averaged over an 8-hour workshift) for inorganic arsenic compounds.

DEFICIENCY MAY CAUSE OR BE ASSOCIATED WITH:

Disorders of heart and skeletal muscle, low serum arsenic are correlated with central nervous system disorders, vascular disease and cancer.

THERAPEUTIC USES

Altered methionine metabolism, haemodialysis, pro-myelocytic leukaemia (as medical treatment not as a nutritional item).

SAFE DAILY DOSAGE

12-25 µg/day

TOXICITY

Despite arsenic's reputation as a poison, it actually has fairly low toxicity in comparison with some other metals, although with chronic exposure there is some concern about arsenic's effect on chromosomes and its carcinogenicity.

Organic forms of arsenic as found in foods are relatively safe.

Inorganic or elemental forms of arsenic can accumulate in the body. The various oxidised forms of arsenic can also have toxicity problems.

The inorganic form of arsenic is more toxic than organic forms and arsenite (3+) [arsenic trioxide (As_2O_3)] is more toxic than arsenite (5+) e.g. arsenic trioxide causes skin and lung cancer, and may cause internal cancers such as liver, bladder, kidney, colon, and prostate cancers.

Toxic dose: (immediately dangerous to life or health) = 5 mg As/m³ (for all inorganic arsenic compounds).

1 to 2.5 mg/kg body weight of arsenic trioxide is a potentially fatal dose.

0.3% of the population have elevated arsenic hair levels.

SYMPTOMS

Anorexia, acute respiratory distress syndrome (ARDS), dermatosis, depletes body's store of phosphate, bladder cancer, cerebral oedema, confusion, coughing, dimness of vision, diplopia, diarrhoea, fatigue, gastroenteritis, haematopoiesis, increased capillary permeability, depression, hallucinations, hair loss, headache, heart disease, hyperkeratosis of palms and soles, jaundice, kidney damage, liver damage, loss of pain sensation, lung cancer, muscle weakness and pain, multiple organ damage, nausea, peripheral neuritis, respiratory failure due to weakness of the respiratory muscles, sensory disturbance, sensory motor polyneuropathy, skin cancer, tachycardia.

Chronic Exposure

Chronic exposure is characterized by malaise, peripheral sensorimotor neuropathy, anaemia, jaundice, gastrointestinal complaints, and characteristic skin lesions including hyperkeratosis (small corn-like elevations) and hyperpigmentation. Hyperkeratosis usually appears on the palms or soles.

Pigmentation changes and hyperkeratosis can take 3 to 7 years to appear.

Chronic inhalation can also lead to conjunctivitis, irritation of the throat and respiratory tract, and perforation of the nasal septum.

Chronic exposure can cause allergic contact dermatitis.

Chronic exposure may be more serious for children because of their potential longer latency period.

Population at Risk of Toxicity

Those exposed to weed killers, insecticides, fumes from burning arsenic containing coals and oils e.g. miners, smelter workers, vineyard workers.

TREATMENT

Vitamin C, EDTA chelation, dimercaprol.

Cadmium (Cd)

SOURCE

Air pollution, cigarette smoke, contaminated seafood, soft water, pesticides, phosphate fertilisers, galvanised pipes, rubber tyres, solders, urban sewerage sludge, oysters (contaminated), potatoes.

Spinach, peanuts and cauliflower concentrate cadmium. High grain-fibre diets are associated with higher intake of cadmium.

Acid soils increase uptake of cadmium by vegetables.

OCCUPATIONAL EXPOSURE

Mines, zinc smelters, refiners of metals, plants that make cadmium products such as batteries (nickel–cadmium), coatings or plastics (cadmium stearate – plastic stabiliser).

Blood-cadmium concentration of smokers is 1-4 µg/l, which is 5 times higher than non-smokers.

0.8% of the population have elevated body burden of cadmium.

UPTAKE INCREASED IN:

Deficiency of vitamin D, copper, iron, calcium and zinc; multiple pregnancies, post menopausal women.

Iron deficiency increases absorption of cadmium, lead, and aluminum.

ABSORPTION

5% of oral dose

50% of inhaled dose

ANTAGONISTS

Vitamin C, calcium, eggs, garlic, high protein diets, iron, lipoic acid, methionine, onion, pectin, quercetin, selenium, zinc, glutathione.

MECHANISM OF TOXICITY

Interacts with calcium in the skeletal system to produce osteodystrophies, replaces zinc on metallothionein, competes with zinc for binding sites in various enzymes and proteins, impairs regulation of calcium and phosphorus balance in the body, reduces calcium incorporation in bones, induces DNA strand breaks and chromosomal aberration, increases oxidant stress, inhibits sulfhydryl containing enzymes, interferes with cellular Na+/K+ pumps, depresses levels of noradrenalin, serotonin and acetylcholine; depletes glutathione and protein bound sulfhydryl groups, suppresses apoptosis of cells, carcinogenic, immunotoxic, reduces collagen production in bones, impedes alkaline phosphatase activity, thus impairing bone formation.

Cadmium is a cumulative toxin.

SYMPTOMS OF TOXICITY

Aggression, alopecia, anaemia, anosmia, bone fractures, cancer (prostate, bladder, lung, liver), chronic bronchitis, decreased verbal intelligence, difficulty in walking, fatigue, hypertension, irritable gut, increases blood pressure, increased renin activity, kidney and liver damage, nephrotoxic, lower back pain, protein and sugar in urine, pulmonary emphysema, osteoporosis, reduction in growth, renal stones, scaly, dry skin and yellow teeth.

MAXIMUM SAFETY DOSE

70 μg/day

Provisional weekly tolerable intake for cadmium is 7 μg/kg/week.

Note: More cadmium is absorbed if the diet is low in calcium, protein or iron.

Diabetics are more prone to experience the negative effects of cadmium.

TOXIC DOSE

200-390 μg/day

HALF LIFE IN BODY

Elimination half life	10-30 years

EXCRETION

An excretion rate of 2-3 μg Cd/g creatinine is associated with a 10% probability of renal tubular dysfunction.

Fluorine (F)

STORED IN:
Bone, kidney, liver.

Fluorine is highly reactive and the most chemically unstable of all the halogens. It is not found by itself, but reacts violently with most elements to become a fluoride.

SOURCE
Artificially fluoridated water, calf liver, mackerel, salted pork, sardines, sea salt, sunflower seeds, beans and peas, legumes, tea.

Toothpaste. Average fluoride content in a tube is 1100 ppm or 1mg/gm.

Fluorine is a common ingredient in anaesthetics, hypnotics, psychiatric drugs, military nerve gas (Soman) and prozac (fluoxetine HCl)

PROCESSING LOSSES
Tends to be concentrated with processing.

FUNCTIONS FACILITATED
Acts locally as an antibiotic, killing oral bacteria associated with caries; immobilises calcium and magnesium, increases bone mass but not strength, replaces bicarbonate in bone.

DEFICIENCY MAY CAUSE OR BE ASSOCIATED WITH:
None recorded.

THERAPEUTIC USES
Dental caries.

Recent evidence suggests limited application in these symptoms only if applied topically – acts as an antibiotic.

DAILY DOSAGE	
SR	0.3-1.0 mg

Children under the age of 12 months should not be exposed to fluoridated water.

Age of Child	Average Weight*	Milligrams of Fluoride Capable of Producing symptoms
2 years	~12 kg	1.2 - 3.6 mg
3 years	~15 kg	1.5 - 4.5 mg
4 years	~16 kg	1.6 - 4.8 mg
5 years	~18 kg	1.8 - 5.4 mg
6 years	~20 kg	2.0 - 6.0 mg
7 years	~22 kg	2.2 - 6.6 mg
8 years	~25 kg	2.5 - 7.5 mg
9 years	~28 kg	2.8 - 8.4 mg

EFFECTS OF OVERDOSAGE AND TOXICITY

Increases risk of: iodine deficiency, osteosarcoma, dental fluorosis, and enamel dystrophy.

Excess accumulation occurs in teeth, cartilage, tendons, blood vessel walls and bones in proportion to the level and duration of fluoride intake.

Acute	**(0.1-8mg/F/kg body weight)** Abdominal cramps (53%), gastrointestinal pain, diarrhoea (65%), nausea (97%), vomiting (68%), headaches (14%), fatigue (4%), gastric ulcers, loss of appetite (13%), itching (9%), weakness (10%), numbness and tingling of extremities (4%), profuse sweating (12%). All the above symptoms and percentages are from records of patients who experienced the effects of municipal water supply being hyper fluoridated.
Chronic	**(>5-10mg/day)** Birth defects, bone abnormalities, bone cancer, calcification of ligaments, damages surface of gastric mucosa, fluoride hypersensitivity, lowers IQ, mottled teeth or fluorosis, osteosclerosis, exostosis of the spine, still births and early infant mortality (based on fluoridated areas in India).
Sublethal	**(>40mg/day)** Gastrointestinal symptoms, weakness.
Lethal	**(>5 mg/kg body weight)** Abdominal pains, diarrhoea, convulsions, excess salivation, nausea, skin rashes.

Melatonin reduces fluorine toxicity

POPULATION AT RISK OF FLUORIDE TOXICITY

Babies, infants, diabetics, athletes, renal patients.

During the first six years of life, the average body weight of a child ranges from 3 to 18 kg (average weight is 12 kg over this period). It is estimated that the child will drink one litre of fluid per day at a fluoride concentration of 1 ppm, equivalent to 1 mg of fluorine per day. For a 12 kg child, this is equivalent to an intake of 0.08mg/kg body weight/day, for an adult of 70 kg it will be 0.014 mg/kg body weight/day. In other words, the child will receive a 7 fold increase in fluoride exposure compared to an adult. The child dose is close to the toxic dose of 0.1 mg/kg body weight.

TECHNICAL NOTES

SYNERGISTIC NUTRIENTS

Glutathione, calcium, iodine and vitamin C reduce toxicity of fluoride.

Iron, magnesium, molybdenum may reduce fluoride toxicity.

Fluoride salts
Sodium fluoride is an experimental tumourigenic and teratogen.

It is produced as a hazardous waste by-product from manufacturers of aluminium. It is a common ingredient in rat and cockroach poisons.

Symptoms of toxicity include: burning, itching, prickly skin, drooping eyelids, tremors, muscle weakness, headache, cyanosis, nausea, vomiting and salivary gland changes.

Potassium fluoride is more toxic than sodium fluoride.

Aluminium and Fluoride:

Cooking in aluminium pots with fluoridated water concentrates aluminium to 600 ppm, where as water without fluoride did not.

The aluminium fluoride that is formed crosses the blood brain barrier with ease and may be the cause of Alzheimer's disease reported with aluminium toxicity.

ENZYME SYSTEMS INVOLVED

Activates: Amylase and adenyl cyclase.

Inactivates: Cholinesterase, DNA nucleases, enolase, hyaluronidase, phosphoglucomutase and phosphatase.

Lead (Pb)

SOURCE

General diet 60-90 µg/day.

Atmospheric pollution, bone meal, canned tuna, cigarette smoke, canned fish, house dust, inner city urban environments, lead based paint, lead plumbing, motor car exhausts, painted toys, vegetation along roadsides.

Concentrates in: Brussel sprouts, spinach, broccoli, cucumbers and wine.

OCCUPATIONAL EXPOSURE

Battery plants, bottle cap makers, canners, explosive makers, plumbers, pottery workers, smelters, soldering, typesetters.

SUSCEPTIBILITY INCREASED IN:

Children, nursing mothers, zinc deficiency, magnesium deficiency.

Iron deficiency increases absorption of cadmium, lead, and aluminum.

Approximately 3% of the population have high body burdens of lead.

ANTAGONISTS

Vitamin B complex, B_1, B_3, C, E, calcium, chromium, copper, cysteine, fibre, iron, lipoic acid, lysine, methionine, quercetin, selenium, sulphur, taurine. These nutrients decrease absorption and tissue build up, and protect enzymes. Vitamins B1 & C, protect the reproductive system from lead-induced cellular apoptosis.

FOODS THAT REDUCE TOXICITY

Citrus products, eggs, garlic, onion, wheat germ.

MECHANISM OF TOXICITY

Alters cell permeability, acts as a clastogen, calcium, iron and zinc deficiency enhances lead toxicity by increasing absorption of toxic metals and by exchanging with essential minerals on biochemical active sites, including receptor proteins in the brain; induces direct DNA damage, inhibits DNA synthesis and repair, inhibits gamma – amino levulinic acid dehydrase and ferro chelatase, inhibits sulfhydryl groups, interferes with haemoglobin synthesis, interacts with calcium in the nervous system to impair cognitive development, replaces zinc on heme enzymes and zinc proteins, hinders the activity of zinc, vitamin B_1 and magnesium; induces oxidative stress.

SYMPTOMS OF TOXICITY

Anaemia, anorexia, anxiety, behavioural abnormalities, cognitive impairment, confusion, constipation, coordination problems, depression, dizziness, drowsiness, fatigue, headaches, kidney damage, peripheral neuropathy, pain in muscle and bones, restlessness, tremors, low IQ, hyperactivity, impulsivity, juvenile delinquency, violent behaviour.

SAFE MAXIMUM EXPOSURE RANGE	
Children	0.6-10 µg
Pregnant women	10-78 µg

BLOOD TOXICITY LEVEL
>25 µg/l

STORED IN:

Bones, liver.

Mercury (Hg)

SOURCE

Body talcs and powders, contaminated seafood, cosmetics, dental amalgam, grains treated with fungicides, fabric softeners, fungicides used on lawns, trees and shrubs; haemorrhoid suppository preparations, mercury treated seeds, mercurochrome, pesticides, photo engraving, wood preservatives, large fish, thimerosal (mercury based preservative used in vaccines).

OCCUPATIONAL EXPOSURE

Battery makers, boilermakers, dental nurses, dentists, electroplaters, lamp makers, mirror makers, paint makers, seed handlers, textile printers, thermometer makers.

TOXICITY SUSCEPTIBILITY INCREASED IN:

Babies, foetus, pregnant women, underweight infants, zinc and cadmium overload.

0.1% of the population have elevated mercury levels.

ANTAGONISTS

Vitamins C, B_5, B_{12}, alginate, cysteine, glutathione, lipoic acid, methionine, N-acetyl cysteine, pectin, selenium, pyridoxal-5-phosphate.

Vitamin A may help brain function in mercury toxic individuals.

Selenium decreases toxicity by forming selenium-mercury complexes

FOODS THAT REDUCE TOXICITY

Asparagus, brussels sprouts, eggs, garlic, legumes.

MECHANISMS OF TOXICITY

Mercury and methyl mercury induce the production of free radicals, induce the depression of glutathione synthesising enzymes, alters protein structure, binds to proteins and enzymes containing sulfhydryl groups, increases inflammatory cytokines, inhibits insulin production, induces food intolerance to wheat and milk proteins.

SYMPTOMS OF TOXICITY

Acute myocardial infarction, anaemia, anorexia, Asperger's syndrome, autism, ataxia, autoimmune disease, birth defects, brain damage, central nervous system (CNS) disorders, colitis, constriction of visual field, depression, dermatitis, diabetes, distal parasthesia (may involve tongue), dizziness, drowsiness, dysarthria, dyslexia, emotional instability, fatigue, hair loss, headaches, hyperactivity disorders, hypertension, increased oxidation of LDL, insomnia, kidney damage, learning difficulties, loss of appetite, loss of memory, loss of sexual drive and ambition, loss of vision and hearing, mental impairment, metallic taste, multiple sclerosis, nausea, nephrotic syndrome, nervousness, numbness, problems with coordination, psychosis, shyness, thirst, tingling of lips and feet, tremors, weakness.

ACCEPTABLE INTAKE	
Adult	0.1mg/day
Infant	0.1ug/kg body weight

Note: There may be a long latency period between time of exposure and symptoms.

½ life clearance from the body is 70 days.

ENZYMES SYSTEM INHIBITED OR MODULATED

Superoxide dismutase, glutathione peroxidase, xanthine oxidase, cysteine dioxygenase, gamma-glutamyltranspeptidase (GGT), sulfite oxidase, B_6 kinase.

STORED IN:

Bone marrow, brain, kidney (50%), liver, spleen.

Absorbed readily through skin and gastrointestinal tract.

Nickel

At low doses – nickel can act as an essential nutrient

SOURCE

Oatmeal, dried beans, peas, nuts, chocolate, cigarettes.

FUNCTIONS FACILITATED

Binds to chromosomes and ion channels – the effect of this is unknown, influences the production or action of the following hormones – prolactin, adrenaline, noradrenaline and aldosterone; maintains cGMP signalling, may improve cardiovascular health.

The enzyme urease is a nickel metalloenzyme. This enzyme can be a major virulence factor for the human gastric pathogen Helicobacter pylori.

DEFICIENCY MAY CAUSE OR BE ASSOCIATED WITH:

Abnormal bone growth, altered metabolism of calcium, vitamin B_{12} and energy nutrients; low blood glucose levels, increased blood pressure, low sperm count and decreased number of mobile sperm.

DAILY DOSAGE	
Daily dietary intake	69-169 µg

TOXIC DOSE
>60 mg/day

ENVIRONMENTAL EXPOSURE

Dental or orthopaedic implants, inexpensive jewellery, jewellery, nickel coins, nickel/cadmium batteries.

TOXICITY

Toxicity varies widely depending on chemical forms.

Nickel toxicity is associated with: oxidation of tissue (i.e. damaged chromosomes), altered hormone and enzyme activity, poor immunity, poor regulation of the movement of ions through the cell membrane (the end result being poor glucose regulation), blood pressure abnormalities, poor growth rates, tissue magnesium deficiency, accumulation of iron or zinc.

Nickel can act as a carcinogen.

ANTAGONISTS

Calcium, iron, magnesium, phytates, zinc.

All these affect absorption of nickel from the gut.

TOXIC SYMPTOMS

Apathy, asthma, allergic contact dermatitis, cyanosis, diarrhoea, dyspnoea, fever, headaches, insomnia, nausea, skin allergies, tachypnoea, vomiting.

STORED IN

Lungs, kidneys and some hormone producing tissues.

APPENDIX

VITAMIN SYNONYMS

A1 - Retinol

B1 - Thiamine, Thiamin hydrochloride, Thiamine chloride, Thiamini Hydrochloridum, Thiamini chloridum, Aneurine hydrochloride

B2 - Riboflavin, Vitamin G

B3 - Niacin, Nicotinic Acid

B4 - Adenine

B5 - Pantothenic Acid

B6 - Pyridoxine, Adermine hydrochloride, Piridossina cloridrato, Pyridoxinii chloridum, Pyridoxini hydrochloridum, Pyridoxinium chloride, Pyridoxol hydrochloride

B8 - Folic acid

B12 - Cobalamin, Cyanocobalamin, Hydroxocobalamin

B15 - Pangamic Acid plus Thiamine

B17 - Laetrile, Amygdalin

Bc - Folic acid, Pteroylglutamic acid

Bt - Carnitine, Levocarnitine

Bx - p-Aminobenzoic acid

C - Ascorbic Acid

D2 - Ergocalciferol, Calciferol, Ergocalciferolum, Irradiated Ergosterol, Viosterol

D3 - Cholecalciferol

E - Tocopherol

F - Essential Fatty Acids belonging to the linoleic acid family

G - Riboflavin, Riboflavinium, Lactoflavin, Vitamin B(2)

H - Biotin, Coenzyme R

K1 - Phytomenadione, Phytonadione, Methylphytylnaphthochinonum, Phylloquinone, Phytomenad

K2 - Menaquinone

K3 - Mendione, Menadionum, Menaph, Menaphthene, Menaphthone, Methylnaphthochinonum

L - Vitamin L1, gamma-Amino benzoic acid

M - Folic acid

P - Rutin, Bioflavonoids, Citrus Flavonoid compounds

PP - Nicotinamide, Niacinamide, Nicotinamidum, Nicotylamide, Nicotinic acid amide

Q - Pyrroloquinoline Quinone

T - Tegolin, Termitin, Torutilin, Temina, Factor T

U - 3-amino-3-carboxypropyl dimethysulfonium Cl or Br S-methyl methionine

CHAPTER 6

Disease and Nutrient Requirements

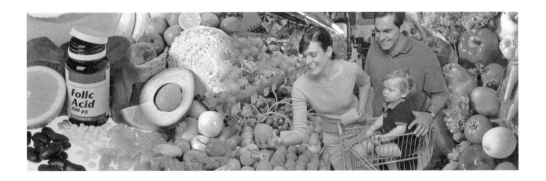

Condition or Symptom	Nutrient
Abnormally high body weight	B1, carnitine, CLA, calcium, CoQ10
Acetaminophen overdose	Cysteine, lipoic acid, SAMe, glutathione, N-acetyl-cysteine
Achlorhydria	B12, iron, zinc, histidine, Betaine HCL, pepsin
Acne	Biotin, zinc, B5, A
Acne rosacea	A, B2
Acne vulgaris	A, B12, Folic Acid, zinc, B5
Acute hearing loss	Co Enzyme Q10
Acute leukaemia	A, D, K
Adeno-carcinoma of the stomach	B3, selenium, C
Addiction	Tyrosine, dl-phenylalanine, tryptophan, acetyl-l-carnitine, NAD, magnesium, adenosine, valine
Adrenal stress	B5, C, potassium, magnesium, copper, tyrosine
Ageing or elderly individuals	E, Folic Acid, K, B1, B2, B3, glutathione, cysteine, glutamine, acetyl-l-carnitine, selenium, silicon, carnosine, leucine, proline, threonine, phosphatidylserine, pepsin, n-acetyl-cysteine, r-lipoic acid, copper, resveratrol
Agitation or aggression	Phenylalanine, tryptophan, selenium, B12, DHA/EPA
Agitated Depression	Alanine, tryptophan
Agrophobia	Inositol, tryptophan, magnesium
AIDS	A, B1, Co Enzyme Q10, carnitine, cysteine, glutamine, glutathione, Tryptophan, methionine, selenium, n-acetyl-cysteine, r-lipoic acid
Air pollution exposure	Beta- Carotene, E, selenium, methionine, glutathione, r-lipoic acid, molybdenum
Alcohol withdrawal	B1, dl-phenylalanine, taurine, tryptophan, tyrosine, magnesium
Alcoholism	B1, B2, B3, B5, B12, Biotin, C, Choline, Essential Fatty Acids, Folic Acid, Arginine, glutamine, glutathione, methionine, magnesium, potassium, selenium, zinc, inositol, pepsin, SAMe, GLA, molybdenum, valine, taurine, carnitine
Allergic conjunctivitis	Bioflavonoids
Allergies	B5, B6, B12, Bioflavonoids, C, Essential Fatty Acids, cysteine, Histidine, magnesium, manganese, pancreatic enzymes, GLA, molybdenum
Allergic uretheritis	Adenosine, zinc, C

Condition or Symptom	Nutrient
Alopecia	Biotin
Alzheimer's disease	Choline, Co Enzyme Q10, E, Tocotrienols, K, acetyl-l-carnitine, NAD, Adenosine, tyrosine, carnosine, phosphatidylserine, r-lipoic acid, resveratrol, DHA/EPA, copper
Amenorrhoea	Carnitine
Amblyopia	B2, B12
Amyotrophic lateral sclerosis	Threonine, creatine, n-acetyl-cysteine
Anaemia (microcytic)	B6, C, Folic Acid, iron, B12, histidine, copper, zinc
Anaemia (megoblastic)	B12
Angina	Co Enzyme Q10, E, Essential Fatty Acids, resveratrol, dimethyl-glycine, bromelain, selenium, lysine, proline, magnesium, carnitine, B12, pyridoxal-5-phosphate
Angiogenic disorders – tumour growth diabetic retinopathy	Tocotrienols
Anorexia	B12, carnitine, zinc, tryptophan, pancreatic enzymes
Anthracycline chemotherapy drug (doxornbicin) therapy	Co Enzyme Q10
Anti-convulsant medication use	Biotin, folate
Anurism	Copper, C, glycine, lysine, proline
Anxiety	B3, B6, NAD, magnesium, histidine, taurine, tryptophan, zinc, SAMe, inositol, calcium
Apathy	B12, B3
Aphthous stomatitis	Folic Acid, B12
Arrhythmia	Co Enzyme Q10, carnitine, magnesium, adenosine, taurine
Arteriosclerosis	C, K, magnesium, glycine , proline, lysine, zinc, silicon, resveratrol
Arthritis	A, B2, B3, B5, B6, B12, Bioflavonoids, D, E, glutathione, glucosamine n-acetyl-glucosamine, glycine, C, DHA/EPA, calcium, copper, silicon, manganese, zinc, bromelain, boron, histidine, lysine, pancreatic enzymes
Asthma	A, B5, B6, Bioflavonoids, magnesium, DHA/EPA, carnitine, glutathione, Alpha-ketoglutarate, molybdenum, manganese, taurine, r-lipoic acid
Asthma- exercised induced	C, magnesium
Astrocytoma	D, K
Ataxia	Choline

Condition or Symptom	Nutrient
Atherosclerosis	B3, B6, Beta-Carotene, Bioflavonoids, C, Choline, Co Enzyme Q10, E, Tocotrienols, Folic Acid, arginine, glutathione, dimethyl-glycine, Bromelain, magnesium, manganese, methionine, proline, iodine, r-lipoic acid, resveratrol, DHA/EPA , copper, silicon, taurine, quercetin
Athletes	C, bioflavonoids, lysine, proline, glycine, zinc, creatine, bromelain, leucine, Isoleucine, methionine
Athletic performance	B6, alanine, aspartate, asparagines, creatine, carnosine, alpha-ketoglutarate, glycine, lysine, valine
Atrophic gastritis	B12, digestive enzymes
Attention Deficit Disorders (ADHD)	B12, glutamine, iron, dimethyl-glycine, folate, SAMe acetyl-l-carnitine, DHA, GLA, lactobacillus, B12, carnosine, folacin
Autism	A, B6, glutamine, carnosine, dimethyl-glycine, folacin, methylcobolamin, SAMe, Vitamin D, folate, carnosine
Autoimmune disease	A, D, E, glycine, glucosamine, n-acetyl-glucosamine, DHA/EPA
Autoimmune encephalomyelitis	D, phosphatidylserine
Autonomic dysfunction	B1, B5
Back Pain	Calcium, glycine, lysine, proline, vitamin C, glucosamine, copper, chondroitin sulphate
Bayler's disease (intrahepatic cholestasis)	E, lactobacillus, fibre
Bell's palsy	Lysine
Behavioural disturbance	Serine, zinc, tryptophan, DHA/EPA
Benign prostatic hyperplasia	Essential Fatty Acids, zinc, glycine
Benzene exposure	A, glutathione
Beriberi	B1
Biliary obstruction or atresia	K, A,D,E, leucine, MCT oil, SAMe
Biopterin substitution	Folic Acid, C
Biotinidase deficiency	Biotin
Bladder cancer– reduces risk of	C
Bladder cancer– stage II	B6
Bladder or bowel incontinence	B12
Bleeding gums	Bioflavonoids, C, copper, rutin
Blood clots	E, C, bromelain, DHA/EPA
Blurred vision	B2
Bone fractures	A, C, D, aspartate, glutamine, calcium, lysine, glycine, proline, rutin, chondroitin sulphate

Condition or Symptom	Nutrient
Breast hyperplasia	Iodine
Breast Cancer – stage II	B6
Brittle nails	A, Biotin, calcium, iron, silicon
Bronchial asthma	B12, Co Enzyme Q10, magnesium, DHA/EPA, quercetin
Bronchitis	A, cysteine, bromelain, zinc, manganese, n-acetylcysteine
Broncho pulmonary dysplasia	E
Bruising	Bioflavonoids, K, C, bromelain
Burning leg or feet syndrome	B5, B1, biotin
Burning legs	Biotin
Burning Mouth Syndrome	Iron, zinc, B complex
Burns	B3, Bioflavonoids, C, E, Essential Fatty Acids, arginine, cysteine, biotin, Methionine, chloride, potassium, zinc
Burns and scalds	Biotin, A, E, methionine, zinc
Bursitis	B12, C, bromelain, Chondroitin sulphate, magnesium
Cachexia	Co Enzyme Q10, carnitine, glutathione, DHA/EPA, r-lipoic acid, pancreatic Enzymes, NAD
Calcium bone spurs	B12, magnesium
Calcium kidney stones	K, magnesium
Cancer: These selection of nutrients basically apply to all cancers	A, B3, Beta-Carotene, Bioflavonoids, C, choline, carnitine, glycine, lysine, D3, Quercetin, bromelain , digestive enzymes, lactobacillus, MCT oil, fish oil, proline, resveratrol
	Mitochondrial nutrients: tocopheryl succinate, acetyl-l-carnitine, CoQ10, lipoic acid, NAD, K
Cancer – Basal cell carcinoma	Selenium, creatine
Cancer – Bladder	B6, C, selenium, B6, genistein, Lactobacillus
Cancer – brain	D3, K2, K3, quercetin, CLA, alpha carotene GLA, mitochondrial nutrients
Cancer – Breast	A, B6, D, Co Enzyme Q10, Tocotrienols, indole-3-carbinol, genistein, limonene Pyridoxal-5-phosphate, C, conjugated linoleic acid (CLA), lactobacillus, molybdenum, selenium, d-glucaric acid, bromelain, DHA/EPA
Cancer – Cervical	C, Co Enzyme Q10, indole-3-carbinol, B6, resveratrol, pyridoxal-5-phosphate, Tocopheryl succinate, folate, B12
Cancer – Colon	Choline, calcium, fibre, lactobacillus, selenium, D-glucaric acid, D3, A, C, modified citrus pectin, genistein, CLA , B12, resveratrol
Cancer – Colorectal	C,D3, as above

Condition or Symptom	Nutrient
Cancer – Endometrial	C, B6
Cancer – Leukemia	A, K, D3,B6, E, C, genistein, adenosine, creatine, quercetin, lycopene, resveratrol
Cancer – Liver	Choline, Tocotrienols, selenium, alpha carotene, creatine, SAMe, EPA, Limonene, GLA, B12, Carnitine
Cancer – Lung	C,D3, A, B6, Co Enzyme Q10, selenium, alpha-carotene
Cancer – Lymphoma	A, C
Cancer – Melanoma	C, B6, A, D3,quercetin, genistein, apigenin, glycine, selenium, CLA, Resveratrol, tocotrienols
Cancer – Oesophageal	C, molybdenum, lycopene, glutamine, genistein
Cancer – Oral	Beta-Carotene, glutathione, folate, C
Cancer – Osteosarcoma	A, D3, taurine, resveratrol
Cancer – Ovarian	Bromelain, A, quercetin, genistein, folic acid, resveratrol
Cancer – Pancreatic	Co Enzyme Q10, methionine, selenium, C, D- limonene, resveratrol, Pyridoxal-5-phosphate
Cancer – Prostate	A, C,D3, Co Enzyme Q10, selenium, zinc, indole-3-carbinol, lycopene Quercetin, tocopheryl succinate, mitochondrial nutrients, modified citrus pectin, CLA, genistein, resveratrol
Cancer – Salivary glands	C
Cancer – Skin	Tocotrienols, selenium, alpha carotene,B3, GLA
Cancer – Stomach	C, molybdenum, lycopene, genistein, glutathione
Cancer – Uterine	A, folic acid
Cancer therapy (tocopheryl succinate form)	E
Cancers – renal	Molybdenum, alpha-ketoglutarate, C, D3, E, mitochondrial nutrients
Carbon-tetrachloride exposure	Arginine, betaine, pyrrolquinoline quinone
Carcinogen exposure	Choline
Cardiomyopathy	E, selenium, Coenzyme Q10, carnosine , copper, taurine, resveratrol
Cardiovascular disease	B12, Beta-Carotene, Bioflavonoids, B6, carnitine, proline glycine, lysine, Arginine, carnosine, E, genistein, copper, K2, resveratrol
Cardiac surgery	Arginine, aspartate, C, CoQ10, C, quercetin, magnesium, taurine. Copper, vitamin K2

Condition or Symptom	Nutrient
Carpal tunnel syndrome	B6
Carpopedal spasm	D, calcium
Cataracts	B2, Bioflavonoids, C, E, taurine, manganese, carnosine, beta-carotene, inositol
Cataracts prevention	A, Beta-Carotene, taurine, manganese, r-lipoic acid
Cerebral ataxia	Carnitine
Cerebral haemorrhage	Bioflavonoids, PQQ, adenosine,K, carnitine
Cerebral palsy	D
Cervical dysplasia	A, C, Folic Acid, indole-3-carbinol
Cheilosis	B2
Chemically sensitive individuals	B6, B12, E, cysteine, glutamine, glutathione, glycine, methionine, taurine
Chemotherapy	Beta-Carotene, cysteine, glutamine, adenosine, CoQ10, malic acid, Resveratrol, mitochondrial nutrients, carnitine
Child birth	K
Cholera patients	B3
Cholestatic liver disease	E, taurine
Cholesterol plaques	Biotin, C, copper, magnesium, taurine
Chorea	Choline
Chromosome breaks	B12
Chronic bronchitis	B5
Chronic fatigue syndrome	B1, Co Enzyme Q10, acetyl-l-carnitine, 5HT, alpha-keto-glutarate, Malic acid, r-lipoic acid, DHA/EPA, lactobacillus, magnesium, methylcobolamin, hydroxycobalamin, serine, tyrosine
Chronic inflammation	B12, DHA/EPA, glycine, D, n-acetyl-glucosamine, quercetin, rutin, proline, hydroxycobolamin, glutathione, C, E
Chronic malnutrition	Co Enzyme Q10, B vitamins, pancreatic enzymes
Chronic obstructive pulmonary disease (COPD)	Co Enzyme Q10, cysteine, glutathione, n-acetyl-cysteine, glycine, carnitine, lipoic acid, antioxidant
Chronic pelvic pain syndrome in men	Bioflavonoids
Chronic renal failure	D, alanine, glycine, arginine, zinc, CoQ10, genistein
Cirrhosis	Carnitine, choline, methionine, zinc, alanine
Coeliac disease	A, B6, B12, D, E, K, carnitine, SAMe, MCT oil, copper
Cognitive deficits	Acetyl-l-carnitine, aspartic acid, B12, glycine, r-lipoic acid

Condition or Symptom	Nutrient
Cognitive impairment or deficits	B12, iodine, iron, glutamine, phosphatidylserine, folate or folacin, Acetyl-l-carnitine, aspartic acid, glycine
Colds	Bioflavonoids, A, C, zinc, lactobacillus, quercetin
Colds conjunctivitis	A
Colitis	K, iron, DHA/EPA, glutamine, glutathione, Chondroitin sulphate, n-acetyl-glucosamine
Compulsive disorder	Tryptophan, histidine
Confusion	B12, B3, B6, magnesium
Congenital atresia (gall bladder)	E, A, D3, K
Congestive heart failure	B1, Co Enzyme Q10, acetyl-l-carnitine, arginine, creatine, selenium, magnesium
Constipation	B1, B5, C, fibre, tryptophan, inositol, lactobacillus, magnesium
Convulsion	D, calcium, manganese
Coordination impairment	B5, B6, valine
Coronary artery disease	B3, potassium, magnesium, chromium, genistein, C, pyridoxal-5-phosphate DHA/EPA, taurine
Coronary thrombosis	C, DHA/EPA, bromelain
Cramps	B3, B5, potassium, magnesium, calcium, sodium
Crohn's disease	A, B2, B6, B12, C, D, Essential Fatty Acids, Folic Acid, K, glutathione, Chondroitin sulphate, MCT oil
Cyclosporine therapy	B6, magensium
Cystic fibrosis	Beta-Carotene, E, K, carnitine, cysteine, taurine, zinc, D-mannose, DHA, MCT oil, pancreatic enzymes, n-acetyl-cysteine, copper
Cystic mastitis	E, GLA
Cystitis	A, D-mannose
Decreased serum potassium	B5
Degenerative diseases	Beta-Carotene
Degenerative vascular disease	C
Dementia	B12, B3, phosphatidylserine, methylcobolamin, r-lipoic acid, copper, carnosine, resveratrol
Demyelination	B5, B12, phosphatidylserine
Depression	C, acetyl-l-carnitine, tryptophan, tyrosine, glutamine, adenosine, Magnesium, selenium, phenylalanine, calcium, SAMe, B12, GLA, Phenylalanine, methylcobolamin, calcium
Dermatitis	Biotin, B3

Condition or Symptom	Nutrient
Detoxification of benzoic acid	B5, glycine
Diabetes	A, B1, B3, B5, Biotin, C, Co Enzyme Q10, E, Essential Fatty Acids, Magnesium, valine, lysine, taurine, leucine, chromium, carnitine, Malic acid, pancreatic enzymes, inositol, DHA/EPA, quercetin
Diabetes (type 1)	A, Biotin, D, glycine, B3, K2, N-acetylcysteine, alpha-keto-glutarate, taurine
Diabetes (type 2)	Biotin, Folic Acid, B12, A, B1, B3, alanine, glutathione, carnitine, Cysteine, zinc, chromium, leucine, lysine, valine, taurine, magnesium, vanadium, carnosine, alpha-keto-glutarate, r-lipoic acid, CLA, C, D, E, K2
Diabetic peripheral neuropathy	Biotin, B1, r-lipoic acid, carnitine, vitamin D, taurine
Diabetic retinopathy	Tocotrienols, Bioflavonoids, taurine, lysine, zinc, alpha-keto-gluterate, rutin
Diarrhoea	A, B1, B2, sodium chloride, fibre, lactobacillus, pancreatic enzymes
Diseases of connective tissues	A, proline, lysine, glycine, n-acetyl-glucosamine, C, zinc
Diverticular disease	Fibre, lactobacillus, glutathione
Dizziness	B12, leucine, isoleucine
Down's Syndrome	B1, Folic Acid, glutathione zinc, iodine, manganese, taurine, tryptophan, selenium, tyrosine, pancreatic enzymes, SAMe, DHA, methylcobolamin, carnitine
Drug toxicity	C, Choline, glycine, antioxidant nutrients, methionine, cysteine, B6, B12, Folate
Dry eyes	A
Dry mouth	C, betaine, xylitol
Dyslexia	A, B6, DHA
Dysmenorrhoea	B6
Dyspermia	Co Enzyme Q10
Eclampsia	Magnesium, zinc, B6, arginine
Eczema	A, B5, Biotin, Essential Fatty Acids, zinc, calcium, dimethyl-glycine, Pancreatic enzymes, Chondroitin sulphate, GLA
Elderly	B1, B2, B6
Elevated blood fats	Essential Fatty Acids, carnitine
Emotional instability	B1, magnesium
Emphysema	Bioflavonoids, carnitine cysteine, copper, Chondroitin sulphate, r-lipoic acid
Endometrial carcinoma- stage II	B6

Condition or Symptom	Nutrient
Endothelial dysfunction	Folic Acid, C, magnesium, glycine, lysine, proline, arginine
Epstein Barr's virus	Bioflavonoids, quercetin
Epilepsy	B6, Biotin, Bioflavonoids, E, glutamine, leucine, zinc, magnesium, Adenosine, glycine, serine, threonine, taurine, dimethyl-glycine, carnitine
Erection problems	Arginine, folic acid, C
Erythropoietic protoporphyria	Beta-Carotene
Exercise induced peroxidation	E
Excessive perspiration	Magnesium, choline, B1, B5
Exposure to pollutants	C, B12, folate, methionine
External scars	C
Eye irritation	A, B2
Facial paralysis	Carnitine
Failure of adrenocorticotropin to induce eosinopenia	B5
Fat malabsorption	Essential Fatty Acids
Fatigue	Co Enzyme Q10, Folic Acid, methionine, alpha-keto-glutarate, B12, magnesium
Fearfulness with agitation	B1
Fevers	B1
Fibro cystic breast disease	A, E, iodine
Fibromyalgia	Bioflavonoids, B12, tryptophan, malic acid, SAMe, serine
Fluid retention	B5
Folate inhibitory drug use	Folic Acid
Fractures	C
Friedreich's ataxia	Co Enzyme Q10, zinc
Frost bite	Bioflavonoids
Functional psychosis	B12
Fungal Infections (athlete's foot)/ nail fungal infections	A
Gall bladder (congenital atresia)	E, choline
Gall bladder disease	Essential Fatty Acids, choline, E, A, D, K, taurine
Gall bladder stones	Choline, magnesium
Gastrointestinal bleeding	Isoleucine
Gastric ulcers	Co Enzyme Q10, glutamine, glucosamine

Condition or Symptom	Nutrient
Genetic abnormalities	Folic Acid
GENETIC DISEASES	
- Sub acute necrotizing encephalopy	B1
- Leigh's Disease	B1
- Maple syrup disease	B1
- Hyperalanemia	B1
- Lactic acidosis associated with pyruvate deficiency	B1
Geographic tongue	B2
Gingivitis	Co Enzyme Q10
Glaucoma	Bioflavonoids, Choline, GLA
Gliomas	C, D, K, genistein
Glossitis	B6
Glucocorticoid use – long term	Tocotrienols
Gout	Folic Acid, glycine, copper, quercetin
Graft rejection	D
Growth retardation	B5, zinc, alpha-keto-glutarate
Gut trauma or infections	A, arginine, zinc, glutamine, fibre, lactobacillus
Haemorrhages	Bioflavonoids, C,K, bromelain
Haemorrhagic shock	Co Enzyme Q10
Haemorrhoids	Bioflavonoids, rutin, copper, fibre
Heavy metal toxicity	Cysteine, histidine, lysine, selenium, r-lipoic acid, quercetin, glutathione
Hair dryness	B5
Hair loss	B5, lysine, inositol, biotin, silicon
Hand numbness	B6
Hartnup's disease	B3
Headaches	B2, C, Choline, magnesium, adenosine, dimethyl-glycine
Heart disease	C, E, Essential Fatty Acids, acetyl-l-carnitine, magnesium, taurine, copper
Heart failure	Co Enzyme Q10, proline, taurine, magnesium, carnitine, r-lipoic acid, Pyridoxal-5-phosphate, inositol, lactobacillus, copper
Hearing loss	Magnesium, CoQ10, zinc, DHA/EPA, copper

Condition or Symptom	Nutrient
Hepatic encephalopathy	Aspartate, acetyl-l-carnitine, glutathione, alpha-keto glutarate, taurine, valine
Hepatitis	Glutathione, glycine, leucine, valine, taurine, betaine, dimethyl-glycine, Pancreatic enzymes, malic acid, SAMe, carnitine
Hereditary sideroblastic anemia	B6
Herpes	Bioflavonoids, lysine, quercetin, zinc, C
Herpes zoster (shingles)	B12, E, quercetin
High blood cholesterol	B3, C, Choline, alanine, tocotrienols, proline, copper, bromelain, fibre, methionine, taurine, chromium, CoQ10, inositol, biotin, silicon, magnesium
High blood histamine	C
High blood pressure	Bioflavonoids, histidine, C, taurine, bromelain, magnesium, CoQ10, Quercetin, silicon, tryptophan, calcium, zinc, Chondroitin sulphate, Glutathione, genistein, copper, taurine
High LDL levels	Beta-Carotene, copper, magnesium
High protein-oedema	Bioflavonoids, quercetin
HIV infections	Co Enzyme Q10, Beta-Carotene, carnitine, cysteine, tryptophan, selenium, glutathione, glutamine
Hodgkin's disease	A, B3
Homocystinuria	B6, B12, serine, betaine, folate, folacin, methyl-cobolamin
Huntington's disease	Choline
Hyperactivity	B1, B6, Methylcobolamin, folacin, zinc, copper, iron, calcium
Hyperalaninemia	B1
Hyperglycaemia	C, carnosine, vanadium, isoleucine, leucine, lysine, chromium, copper, biotin, K, taurine
Hyperhomocyst(e)inaemia	Folic Acid, B12, B6, serine, betaine
Hyper kertosis (goose-like bumps on arrm)	A
Hyper-mobility of joints	Proline
Hyperparathyroidism	D, magnesium
Hypertension	B3, C, Choline, Co Enzyme Q10, D, carnitine, glutathione, glutamine, Arginine (for salt sensitive hypertensives), calcium, histidine, taurine, Tryptophan, zinc, selenium, magnesium, potassium, carnosine, silicon, copper, glycine

Condition or Symptom	Nutrient
Hyperthyroidism	B1, Co Enzyme Q10, carnitine, taurine, copper
Hypothyroidism	Tyrosine, iodine, selenium, NAD, zinc
Hypertriglyceremia	B3, DHA/EPA, carnitine, fibre, DHA, copper, biotin, taurine
Hypoglycaemia	B6, alanine, carnitine, chromium, manganese, leucine, isoleucine
Hypoxia	B6, Co Enzyme Q10
Ileitis	B12, hydroxycobalamin
Inborn errors of metabolism	B6
Indigestion	B1, betaine HCL, threonine, digestive enzymes, pepsin
Infant growth	Choline, zinc, chromium, GLA
Infection	B1, B5, B12, Bioflavonoids, C, E, zinc, glutamine, asparagines, molybdenum (yeast and fungal infections), selenium
Infertility	B6, C, E, arginine, carnitine, lysine, taurine, chromium, manganese, molybdenum, zinc, chondroitin sulphate, carnitine, selenium
Inflammation	Bioflavonoids, C, E, bromelain, glycine, histidine, selenium, DHA/EPA, Quercetin, Chondroitin sulphate, r-lipoic acid, glutathione, B12, proline
Inflammatory bowel disease	D, bromelain, tryptophan, glycine, DHA/EPA, fibre, lactobacillus, glutathione
Insomnia	B5, B12, tryptophan, calcium, iron, magnesium, adenosine, inositol, calcium
Insulin resistance	Threonine, chromium, zinc, magnesium, vanadium, MCT oil, r-lipoic acid
Intermittent claudication	E, C, bromelain, zinc, dimethyl-glycine, carnitine
Intrahepatic cholestasis (Bayler's disease)	E
Involuntary eye movements	E
Iron overload	Lipoic acid, quercetin, taurine
Irradiation	Cysteine, glutamine, glutathione, adenosine, glucosamine, Histidine, methionine
Irregular heart beat	Magnesium, adenosine, carnitine
Irritable bowel syndrome (IBS)	Glutamine, glutathione, lactobacillus, fibre, DHA/EPA, lysine, fibre
Irritability	B1, B12, valine, tryptophan, calcium, magnesium

Condition or Symptom	Nutrient
Ischaemic heart disease	Co Enzyme Q10, arginine, carnitine, acetyl-l-carnitine, glycine, magnesium, copper, carnosine
Juvenile arthritis	D
Kerotomalacia	A
Kidney stones	Alanine, magnesium, water, r-lipoic acid, K
Korsakoff's psychosis	B1
Lactation	C, D
Lactic acidosis associated with pyruvate carboxylase deficiency	B1
Lameness	Biotin
Laryngospasm	D, calcium
Lead poisoning	B1, lysine, calcium
Leg cramps	B6, Biotin, magnesium, calcium, potassium
Leaky gut	Glutamine, glutathione, glucosamine, n-acetyl-glucosamine, lactobacillus, silicon
Learning deficits	Iron, acetyl-l-carnitine
Leg ulcers	C, glycine, quercetin, zinc
Lesch-Nyhan disease	Folic Acid
Ligament damage	Lysine, proline, glycine, C, bromelain, silicon
Limb numbness	Calcium
Liver cancer	Choline, Tocotrienols, carnitine, resveratrol
Liver detoxification	A, SAMe, C,E, glutathione, B2, lipoic acid, methionine, taurine
Liver disease	B5, B6, arginine, glutathione, betaine, alpha-keto-glutarate, selenium, creatine, leucine, methionine, threonine, carnosine dimethyl-glycine, SAMe, E, valine, taurine
Long term glucocorticoid use	Tocotrienols
Low bone density	K, calcium, D, zinc, manganese, calcium orotates
Low sperm count	Arginine, zinc
Lowered plasma cholesterol	B5
Loss of smell and taste	Zinc
Lung cancer	C, Co Enzyme Q10, Folic Acid
Lyme disease	D
Lymphoedema	Bioflavonoids, quercetin
Macrosomia (abnormally high body weight)	B1

Condition or Symptom	Nutrient
Macular degeneration	Beta-Carotene, C, E, zinc, carnitine
Mania	Choline, zinc
Maple syrup urine disease (branched-chain aminoacidopathy)	B1
Mastectomy patients	Bioflavonoids, quercetin
Measles	A
Medical drug use – statins, mitochondrial encephalomyopathies	Co Enzyme Q10
Melanoma	Tocotrienols, glycine, C
Memory deficits	B1, B6, Choline, phenylalanine, iodine, magnesium, boron, phosphatidylserine
Memory loss or failure	B12, Folic Acid, B1, acetyl-l-carnitine, NAD, B3, histidine, serine, Magnesium, phosphatidylserine, choline
Meniere's disease	Bioflavonoids, lysine
Menopausal symptoms	Genistein, tryptophan, taurine
Menstrual problems	E, Folic Acid, calcium, iron, boron, zinc, phenylalanine
Mental illness	Folic Acid
Mental retardation	B6
Metabisulphite sensitivity	B12, molybdenum
Metabolic syndrome	B1, MCT oil, zinc, chromium, magnesium, B3, mitochondrial nutrients, resveratrol
Methamphetamine addiction	Acetyl-l-carnitine, dl-phenylalanine, tyrosine, tryptophan
Metastasis	Bromelain, glycine, lysine, proline, quercetin, DHA/EPA, C, selenium, Tocopheryl succinate, A, D3, modified citrus pectin, silicon, resveratrol, zinc, Curcumin, genistein, green tea polyphenols.
Microvarices of the vocal cord	Bioflavonoids
Migraine	Bioflavonoids, B2, Magnesium, adenosine
Mitochondrial disease or failure	B2, B3, NAD, Coenzyme Q10, lipoic acid, carnitine, K, C, alpha-keto-glutarate, creatine
Moodiness	C, B12, tryptophan, chromium, magnesium
Morbid obesity	Co Enzyme Q10, calcium, B1, carnitine, iodine, tyrosine, magnesium
Motoneuron disease	Threonine, glycine, vitamin D, B12, folate

Condition or Symptom	Nutrient
Multiple sclerosis	A, B1, B12, D, E, Essential Fatty Acids, copper, selenium, Threonine, glycine, serine, pancreatic enzymes, phosphatidyl serine, adenosylcobalamin, lipoic acid
Muscle building	Arginine, leucine, isoleucine, valine, zinc, chromium, ornithine, alpha-ketoglutarate, silicon
Muscle cramps	E, calcium, magnesium, potassium, sodium
Muscle weakness	D, isoleucine, leucine, taurine, magnesium, CoQ10, E
Muscular degeneration	Bioflavonoids, leucine, valine, E, B6, carnosine, creatine
Muscular disorder	B6, E, CoQ10
Muscular dystrophy	Co Enzyme Q10, E, creatine, carnitine
Myasthenia gravis	Choline, acetyl-l-carnitine, creatine
Myopia	Folic Acid
Nausea of pregnancy	B6, K, GLA
Neonatal jaundice with phototherapy	B2
Nephrotic syndrome	Essential Fatty Acids, arginine, magnesium, glycine, alanine, Resveratrol, r-lipoic acid, carnitine, taurine, carnosine
Nervousness	B5
Neural tubular defects	Folic Acid, inositol
Neuritis or neuropathy	B1, B3, acetyl-l-carnitine, serine, B5, B12, CoQ10, D, adenosylcobalamin, taurine, biotin, lipoic acid, copper
Neuromuscular dysfunction associated with malabsorption	E, acetyl-l-carnitine
Neuromuscular irritability	D, glycine, r-lipoic acid
Night blindness	A, Beta-Carotene, B2
Night terrors	B3
Nitrate exposure	C
Non-Hodgkin's lymphoma	C
Nose bleeds	Bioflavonoids, C, K, rutin
Numbness in hands and feet	B1, B12, adenosylcobalamin
Nursing mothers	B12
Obsessive compulsive disorder	Histidine, inositol
Obesity	Carnitine, calcium, tyrosine, iodine, fibre, MCT oils, CoQ10, GLA, CLA, D, folacin
Oedema	Quercetin, bromelain
Optic neuritis	A, B3

Condition or Symptom	Nutrient
Oral cancers	Beta-Carotene
Oral leucoplakia	Beta-Carotene
Oral mucosa ulcer	B5
Organic aciduria	Carnitine
Osteoarthritis	B5, C, calcium, glucosamine, B3, DHA/EPA, silicon, bromelain, boron, copper, manganese, proline
Osteomalacia	D
Osteoporosis	C, D, K, lysine, boron, calcium, copper, manganese, magnesium, glucosamine, xylitol, zinc
Ozone exposure	E
Paget's disease	K, silicon
Pain	K, arginine, dl-phenylalanine, tryptophan, lysine, (viral type pain), boron (arthritic pain), SAMe (arthritic pain), Malic acid (musculoskeletal pain)
Pain (traumatic type)	Bioflavonoids, lysine, threonine
Palpitations	B1, magnesium, taurine, calcium
Pancreatic and gall bladder disease	A, D,E. K, taurine, glycine, DHA/EPA, pancreatic enzymes
Pancreatic insufficiency	B12, K, leucine, digestive enzymes, bromelain, bicarbonate
Pancreatitis	Bioflavonoids, leucine, MCT oil, K, pancreatic enzymes
Panic attacks	B5, magnesium, inositol
Parasthesia	B12
Parasympathetic underactivity	B1, Magnesium, tyrosine, B5, acetyl-l-carnitine
Parathyroid hyperplasia	Calcium
Parkinson's disease	B6, C, Co Enzyme Q10, E, glutathione, tyrosine, selenium, methionine, Tryptophan, creatine, adenosine, histidine, leucine, SAMe, Phosphatidylserine, r-lipoic acid, carnitine, copper
Patients on epileptic medication	Folic Acid
Pellagra	B3
Periodontal disease	C, Co Enzyme Q10, K
Peripheral neuropathy	B1, B12
Pernicious anaemia	B12
Personality changes	B5
Perthe's disease	Manganese

Condition or Symptom	Nutrient
Pesticide exposure	Beta-Carotene
Peyronie's disease	Carnitine, E
Photophobia	B2
Photosensitivity	Beta-Carotene
Pica	Iron
Platelet aggregation	E
Pollution exposure	A, lipoic acid, glutathione, zinc, molybdenum, C
Poly cystic ovarian syndrome	Iodine
Polyneuritis	B5, r-lipoic acid
Polyneuropathy	B3, r-lipoic acid
Poor appetite	B1, zinc, B12, DHA/EPA
Poor circulation	B3, carnitine, E, DHA/EPA, bromelain, dimethyl-glycine
Poor concentration	Folacin, mthylcobalamin, SAMe, B6, aspartic acid
Poor co-ordination	B6, valine
Poor Digestion	Digestive enzymes, zinc, histidine, glycine, threonine
Poor immunity	A, B1, B2, B5, E, zinc, alanine, arginine, C, glutamine, glutathione, Adenosine, serine, selenium
Poor libido	Folic Acid, zinc, histidine, phenylalanine, tyrosine
Poor mitochondrial function	K, lipoic acid, NAD, glutathione, carnitine, C, zinc, manganese, CoQ10, Alpha-keto-glutarate
Post ischaemic oedema	Bioflavonoids, quercetin, CoQ10, carnitine
Post partum depression	B12, zinc, B6. (Reduce copper levels)
Post traumatic stress disorder	Tryptophan, 5HT, inositol
Pregnancy	B1, B2, C, K, Choline, D, Folic Acid, calcium, iron, phosphate
Pre-eclampsia	Arginine, B6, magnesium, zinc
Premature infants	C, Folic Acid, E taurine, zinc, copper, iron, inositol, DHA
Premenstrual fluid retention	B6, magnesium
Premenstrual tension	E, tryptophan, tyrosine, potassium, magnesium, B6, GLA
Presentation of neural tube defects	B12
Pressure sores	C
Prickly heat	C
Propionic acidemia	Biotin
Prostatitis or hypertrophy	Bioflavonoids, zinc, alanine, glycine, resveratrol
Protein deficiency and imbalances	B3

Condition or Symptom	Nutrient
Pruritis	A
Psoriasis	A, D, Essential Fatty Acids, cysteine, zinc, Chondroitin sulphate
Psychosis	B3, B12
Pulmonary emphysema	A
Radiation	Beta-Carotene, Co Enzyme Q10, r-lipoic acid, glutamine
Radiation pneumonitis infection	Co Enzyme Q10, r-lipoic acid, glutamine
Radiation sickness	B6, r-lipoic acid
Radiotherapy	Bioflavonoids, r-lipoic acid
Radium treatment	B5
Renal disease or Failure	Carnitine, alanine, glycine, CoQ10, threonine, valine, zinc, histidine, isoleucine, leucine, methionine, genistein, r-lipoic acid, acetyl-l-carnitine, carnosine
Respiratory distress syndrome	E, glycine, glutathione
Restenosis	Folic Acid, magnesium
Restlessness	B12, magnesium
Retinitis	Bioflavonoids, A, taurine
Retinitis pigmentosa	A, Co Enzyme Q10, taurine
Retrolental fibroplasia	E
Reye's syndrome	Carnitine
Rheumatoid arthritis	B5, D, E, Tocotrienols, K, histidine, copper, potassium, selenium, zinc, creatine, bromelain, alpha-ketoglutar-ate, EPA, glutamine
Rhinitis	B5
Rickets	D, calcium, phosphorus
Salicylate sensitivity	Glycine
Salivary gland cancer	C
Schizophrenia	B3, B6, Bioflavonoids, Choline, isoleucine (B3 type), B12, methionine (histidilic type), magnesium, zinc, DHA or EPA, glycine, methylcobalamin, glycine
Seizures in new born	B6, folate, glycine
Senile dementia	B12, carnosine, resveratrol
Sensory neuropathy	Co Enzyme Q10
Sepsis	B12, arginine, cysteine, glutamine, zinc, carnosine, glycine, Isoleucine, valine, copper
Shingles	B12
Sickle cell anaemia	E
Sinusitis	A, Bioflavonoids, E, bromelain

Condition or Symptom	Nutrient
Skin cancer	Tocotrienols
Skin disease	B5, B2, B3, zinc, silicon, selenium
Skin disorders	B2, silicon, EPA, GLA, selenium
Smokers	A, C
Smoking withdrawal	B3
Sore tongue	Iron, B12
Sonophobia	B1
Sprains	Bioflavonoids, quercetin, bromelain, glycine, lysine, proline, silicon
Spider bites	Quercetin, taurine, adenosine, C, DHA/EPA
Spinal curvature	Calcium, melatonin, tryptophan, SAMe, E
Spinal injuries	Glycine, threonine, serine, quercetin, bromelain, B12, silicon
Steatohepatitis	E, fibre, lactobacillus
Stiffness of the hands	B6, copper, magnesium, proline
Stomach cancer	C
Strenuous exercise	C, magnesium, leucine, valine, carnosine
Stress	B2, B6, C, Folic Acid, magnesium, glutamine, acetyl-l-carnitine, tyrosine, Isoleucine, leucine, lysine, magnesium, tryptophan, taurine
Stroke	B2, Bioflavonoids, E carnosine, dimethyl-glycine, glycine, copper, magnesium, potassium, r-lipoic acid, Tocotrienols, K, carnitine, resveratrol
Stroke associated brain damage	Tocotrienols, adenosine, quercetin, C, bromelain, PQQ, r-lipoic acid, magnesium, adenosine
Subacute necrotizing encephalopathy (SNE, Leigh's disease)	B1
Suicidal ideation	Tryptophan, magnesium
Sun burn	C, E, zinc
Sun exposure – low levels	D
Sun sensitivity	B6
Surgery	Beta-Carotene, C, K, glutamine, zinc, isoleucine, lysine, methionine, valine, ornithine, arginine, ornithine
Surgical trauma	Bioflavonoids, arginine
Sympathetic dominance	Choline, B1, B5, acetyl-l-carnitine, copper
Syndrome X	D, chromium, zinc, magnesium, B3
Tachycardia	Adenosine, taurine, magnesium, CoQ10, carnitine

Condition or Symptom	Nutrient
Tardive dyskinesia	Choline, E, leucine, manganese
Tennis elbow	B12, manganese
Tetany	D, magnesium
Thalassemia major	E
Thrombosis	E
Tinnitus	A, manganese
Tobacco smoke exposure	C
Toe and Heal pain	B1
Tooth and gum disorders	A
Tooth decay	Bioflavonoids
Tooth growth	B3
Toxin induced cardio-toxicity	Co Enzyme Q10
Trauma	C, Essential Fatty Acids, carnosine
Traumatic brain injury	B2, B3, adenosine, quercetin, magnesium
Tumour growth	Tocotrienols, selenium, A, glycine, B12
Ulcerative colitis	A, B5, B12, D, Essential Fatty Acids, glutathione, glucosamine, bromelain, Threonine, tryptophan, Chondroitin sulphate
Ulcers (duodenal and gastric)	A, glutamine, glucosamine, glycine (chemically induced ulcers), Histidine, threonine, Chondroitin sulphate
Uraemic patients	B6, histidine, isoleucine, leucine, serine, tryptophan, inositol
Urinary frequency	Magnesium, glycine
UV induced skin tumours	B3, A
Varicose ulcers	B5, C, quercetin, K
Varicose veins	Bioflavonoids, E, C, K2, Copper
Vascular fragility	C
Vegetarians	B12, taurine, zinc, calcium
Ventricular fibrillation	Carnitine, adenosine, magnesium, tyrosine
Vertigo	Magnesium
Babies – Very low birth weight	E
Violent behaviour	B12, tryptophan, DHA/EPA
Viral infection (herpes, Epstein Barr's virus)	Bioflavonoids, quercetin, EPA, zinc, C, A
Viral induced nutrient deficiency	Glutamine, cysteine, tryptophan, selenium, glutathione
Viral meningitis	A, zinc, quercetin

Condition or Symptom	Nutrient
Vitamin D2 toxicity	K
Wernicke-Korsakoff syndrome	B1
Wernicke's encephalopathy	B1
Wilson's disease	Cysteine, molybdenum
Wound healing	A,B5, C, E, zinc, arginine, glutamine, glycine, lysine, proline, leucine, ornithine
Xerophthalmia (dry eyes)	A
Yeast Infection	Zinc, iron, C (lower tissue copper levels)
Zollinger-Ellison syndrome	B12

A complementary text to *The Nutrient Bible 8th edition* is:
The Physician's Handbook of Clinical Nutrition 7th edition.

The Physician's Handbook of Clinical Nutrition

SEVENTH EDITION

Completely Revised, updated and expanded

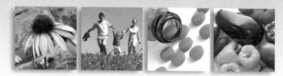

The eagerly-awaited new edition of:
The Physician's Handbook of Clinical Nutrition is finally here!

The Physician's Handbook of Clinical Nutrition is a comprehensive text covering a large number of conditions and nutritional supportive recommendations.

Detailed, practical and easy to use!

- Additional 300 Pages of entirely new material and research
- Contains Tried & Tested Nutritional Treatments
- Up-to-date referencing
- Disease States and Protocols covered in detail
- Cancer Section expanded by 400% & 5 Chapters, incorporating the latest research findings
- Comprehensive Index which takes you straight to the Disease State

This is a must have for any clinician, student or for anyone who strives for optimal health!

ISBN 1-875239-35-9

9 781875 239351

To order a copy of the *Physician's Handbook of Clinical Nutrition 7th edition*, please email: **info@bioconcepts.com.au**

A complementary text to *The Nutrient Bible 8th edition* is:
*The Power of Clinical Nutrition in Cardiovascular
& Respiratory Conditions*

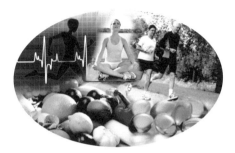

The Power of Clinical Nutrition
in Cardiovascular & Respiratory Conditions

An invaluable new text by leading Clinical Nutritionist
Henry Osiecki & Stephen Eddey

The Power of Clinical Nutrition in Cardiovascular & Respiratory Conditions
comprehensively details the development of many Cardiovascular &
Respiratory Conditions, discusses contributing & risk factors & offers nutritional
recommendations & supplementation options.

It is a practical tool containing comprehensive information on:

- The causes of Cardiovascular Conditions & Atherosclerosis
- Cardiovascular Disorders such as: Angina, Palpitations & Hypertension
- Diet & Exercise for Cardiovascular Conditions
- Risk factors & Treatment options for Sleep Apnoea
- The onset of Asthma & Childhood Asthma Prevention
- Hayfever, Sinusitis & Cystic Fibrosis

*The Power of Clinical Nutrition in Cardiovascular & Respiratory
Conditions:*

- Offers numerous nutritional strategies catered for specific conditions, illnesses &
  diseases
- Extensively profiles many conditions & disease states to explain the reasons
  behind the onset of numerous Cardiovascular & Respiratory Conditions
- Contains over a hundred figures & diagrams illustrating
  various disease processes & showing the overall effect of
  nutritional strategies.

**This is a must have for any clinician, student
or for anyone who strives for optimal health!**

ISBN 978-1-875239-41-2

9 781875 239412

To order a copy of the *The Power of Clinical Nutrition in
Cardiovascular & Respiratory Conditions*, please email:
info@bioconcepts.com.au

A complementary text to *The Nutrient Bible 8th edition* is:
Sleep, Health & Consciousness – A Physician's Guide

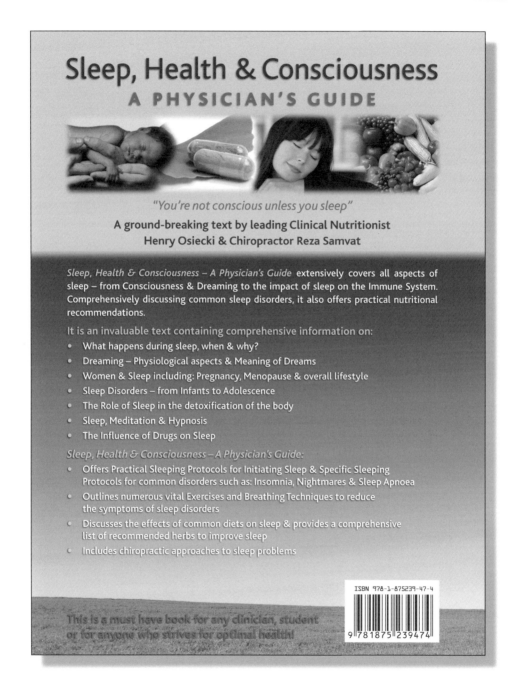

Sleep, Health & Consciousness
A PHYSICIAN'S GUIDE

"You're not conscious unless you sleep"

A ground-breaking text by leading Clinical Nutritionist
Henry Osiecki & Chiropractor Reza Samvat

Sleep, Health & Consciousness – A Physician's Guide extensively covers all aspects of sleep – from Consciousness & Dreaming to the impact of sleep on the Immune System. Comprehensively discussing common sleep disorders, it also offers practical nutritional recommendations.

It is an invaluable text containing comprehensive information on:

- What happens during sleep, when & why?
- Dreaming – Physiological aspects & Meaning of Dreams
- Women & Sleep including: Pregnancy, Menopause & overall lifestyle
- Sleep Disorders – from Infants to Adolescence
- The Role of Sleep in the detoxification of the body
- Sleep, Meditation & Hypnosis
- The Influence of Drugs on Sleep

Sleep, Health & Consciousness – A Physician's Guide:

- Offers Practical Sleeping Protocols for Initiating Sleep & Specific Sleeping Protocols for common disorders such as: Insomnia, Nightmares & Sleep Apnoea
- Outlines numerous vital Exercises and Breathing Techniques to reduce the symptoms of sleep disorders
- Discusses the effects of common diets on sleep & provides a comprehensive list of recommended herbs to improve sleep
- Includes chiropractic approaches to sleep problems

ISBN 978-1-875239-47-4

This is a must have book for any clinician, student or for anyone who strives for optimal health!

9 781875 239474

To order a copy of the ***Sleep, Health & Consciousness –***
A Physician's Guide, please email: **info@bioconcepts.com.au**

Here are further recommended titles by Henry Osiecki which you may find highly beneficial:

- The Physician's Handbook of Clinical Nutrition 7th Edition

- The Power of Clinical Nutrition in Cardiovascular & Respiratory Conditions

- Sleep, Health & Consciousness – A Physician's Guide

- Cancer, Surgery & Radiotherapy CD's

To order your copies of any one of the above titles, please email: **info@bioconcepts.com.au**

Notes